100 Questions & Answers About Your Child's ADHD: From Preschool to College
Second Edition

Ruth D. Nass, MD
Pediatric Neurologist
Child Study Center
Professor of Child Neurology and Child & Adolescent Psychiatry
NYU School of Medicine
New York, NY

Fern Leventhal, PhD
Psychologist
New York State Psychiatric Institute
Assistant Clinical Professor of Medical Psychology (in Psychiatry)
Columbia University
New York, NY

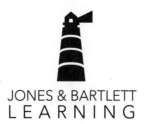

JONES & BARTLETT
L E A R N I N G

World Headquarters

Jones & Bartlett Learning
40 Tall Pine Drive
Sudbury, MA 01776
978-443-5000
info@jblearning.com
www.jblearning.com

Jones & Bartlett Learning
Canada
6339 Ormindale Way
Mississauga, Ontario L5V 1J2
Canada

Jones & Bartlett Learning
International
Barb House, Barb Mews
London W6 7PA
United Kingdom

Jones & Bartlett Learning books and products are available through most bookstores and online booksellers. To contact Jones & Bartlett Learning directly, call 800-832-0034, fax 978-443-8000, or visit our website, www.jblearning.com.

Substantial discounts on bulk quantities of Jones & Bartlett Learning publications are available to corporations, professional associations, and other qualified organizations. For details and specific discount information, contact the special sales department at Jones & Bartlett Learning via the above contact information or send an email to specialsales@jblearning.com.

The authors, editor, and publisher have made every effort to provide accurate information. However, they are not responsible for errors, omissions, or for any outcomes related to the use of the contents of this book and take no responsibility for the use of the products and procedures described. Treatments and side effects described in this book may not be applicable to all people; likewise, some people may require a dose or experience a side effect that is not described herein. Drugs and medical devices are discussed that may have limited availability controlled by the Food and Drug Administration (FDA) for use only in a research study or clinical trial. Research, clinical practice, and government regulations often change the accepted standard in this field. When consideration is given to use of any drug in the clinical setting, the healthcare provider or reader is responsible for determining FDA status of the drug, reading the package insert, and reviewing prescribing information for the most up-to-date recommendations on dose, precautions, and contraindications, and determining the appropriate usage for the product. This is especially important in the case of drugs that are new or seldom used.

Production Credits

Executive Publisher: Christopher Davis
Editorial Assistant: Sara Cameron
Associate Production Editor: Leah Corrigan
Director of Marketing: Alisha Weisman
Manufacturing and Inventory Supervisor: Amy Bacus
Composition: Glyph International

Cover Designer: Carolyn Downer
Cover images: (top) © Edyta Pawlowska/ ShutterStock, Inc.; (bottom left) © Feverpitch/ ShutterStock, Inc.; (bottom right) © Monkey Business Images/ShutterStock, Inc.
Printing and Binding: Malloy, Inc.
Cover Printing: Malloy, Inc.

Library of Congress Cataloging-in-Publication Data
Nass, Ruth D.
  100 questions and answers about your child's ADHD : from preschool to college / Ruth D. Nass and Fern Leventhal.
       p. cm.
  Rev. ed. of: 100 questions & answers about your child's attention deficit hyperactivity disorder. c2005.
  Includes index.
  ISBN 978-0-7637-8179-8 (alk. paper)
  1. Attention-deficit hyperactivity disorder—Popular works. 2. Attention-deficit hyperactivity disorder—Miscellanea. I. Leventhal, Fern. II. Nass, Ruth D. 100 questions & answers about your child's attention deficit hyperactivity disorder. III. Title. IV. Title: One hundred questions and answers about your child's ADHD.

RJ506.H9N37 2011
618.92'8589—dc22
                                          2010018000
6048

Printed in the United States of America
14 13 12 11 10   10 9 8 7 6 5 4 3 2 1

Contents

Preface   v

Introduction   vii

Part 1: The Basics   1

Questions 1–10 address basic concerns about attention deficit hyperactivity disorder (ADHD):
- What is attention deficit hyperactivity disorder (ADHD)?
- Do children outgrow ADHD?
- What parts of the brain are affected in ADHD?

Part 2: Risk Factors, Symptoms, and Diagnosis   15

Questions 11–44 examine symptoms of ADHD and the diagnosis process including:
- What causes ADHD?
- If I have ADHD, will my child also have it?
- Do the symptoms of ADHD change as children mature?

Part 3: Medication and ADHD   49

Questions 45–68 address important issues associated with the medications used to treat and manage ADHD, such as:
- What kinds of medication are used to treat ADHD?
- Can preschoolers take stimulants? Do stimulants affect them differently?
- How do I know the right time to start giving my child ADHD medication? And how long will my child need to stay on stimulants?

Part 4: Negotiating for Academic Success   103

Questions 69–86 review options available to help your child succeed in school:
- What kinds of learning difficulties are commonly associated with ADHD?
- What accommodations should I encourage the school to make for my ADHD child?
- What is an IEP and why do ADHD students need one?

Part 5: Psychosocial Issues   127

Questions 87–100 examine common psychosocial issues children/young adults with ADHD and their families often face, such as:

- How should I talk with my child about an ADHD diagnosis?
- My child's ADHD really has brought anger and frustration into our family life. What can I do?
- Should I let my ADHD teenager drive, knowing that such adolescents have more automobile accidents?

Appendix   143

Glossary   153

Index   159

In 1980, attention deficit disorder (ADD) and attention deficit hyperactivity disorder (ADHD) became the official diagnoses for children with problems of attention and impulsivity, with or without hyperactivity. These behaviors had been labeled "minimal brain dysfunction" in 1960. The change in 1980 clearly reflected a long history of interest and confusion. In the 1970s, as researchers and practitioners began making the connection between daydreaming and the more obvious impulsive and hyperactive behaviors, the diagnostic emphasis began to change. Soon the disorder became widely studied and the treatment widely debated.

Controversy over the diagnosis and treatment of ADHD continues to be in the forefront of the news. Parents can be easily overwhelmed by the amount of information, yet confused about the choices that must be made. ADD and ADHD are serious disorders of childhood and adolescence. If left untreated, they can negatively affect a child's academic functioning, social life, and professional productivity. This book by Drs. Ruth Nass and Fern Leventhal is a welcome compilation of basic knowledge and helpful insights that parents can use to help them through the medical, educational, and social issues that confront them and their children with attention and behavioral problems.

Drs. Nass and Leventhal each have been evaluating children with ADD and ADHD for more than two decades. Ruth Nass, MD, a pediatric neurologist, performs neurological evaluations, makes the diagnosis, and provides medication treatment when indicated. Fern Leventhal, PhD, a pediatric neuropsychologist, administers assessments, exploring children's relative strengths and weaknesses as well as searching for other conditions that commonly co-occur in individuals with ADD and ADHD. In this book, they bring together their separate diagnostic and clinical expertise. Drs. Nass and Leventhal have a gift for communicating information clearly, directly, and sympathetically for the concerned parent. This book is an important resource for families with a child with ADHD. It answers questions they didn't even know they should ask.

Harold Koplewicz, MD
Director of the Nathan Kline Institute for Psychiatric Research
President, Child Study Center Foundation

This book was written to address the many questions that remain unanswered when patients leave our offices. Sometimes there is just not enough time to satisfy the needs of curious, articulate parents. Other times, parents leave our offices, overwhelmed by the diagnosis and unable to put into words the questions that will clarify their misunderstandings and calm their anxieties. In other cases, parents come across magazine articles or hear incomplete information in the media that needs to be simplified or explained. This book provides quick access to that information.

It is our patients, both the parents and the children, who have helped us find the answers to these questions. By trying to appreciate their unique stories, empathize with their problems, and reduce their fears, we have furthered our own knowledge about attention deficit hyperactivity disorder (ADHD). We hope that by reading this book, you too will expand your awareness, information, and understanding of what is happening to your child.

We both would like to acknowledge all the wonderful support we received from our families and friends during the many hours it took to write and edit this book. Without the benefit of their guidance, patience, and love, we never would have gotten through the experience. We would particularly like to thank Ruth's daughter Nora for her photographic contributions and Fern's daughter Emma for her help organizing the valuable resources available in the last section of the book.

There is no doubt that we have been very fortunate to have children of our own who have taught us much about the world and about ourselves. We sincerely hope that you too will listen to your own children, learning what they have to teach you about ADHD and its impact on children and their families. In this way, you can hopefully continue the process that you have already initiated in becoming your child's best advocate.

Fern Leventhal, PhD
Ruth D. Nass, MD

PART ONE

The Basics

What is attention deficit hyperactivity disorder (ADHD)?

Do children outgrow ADHD?

What parts of the brain are affected in ADHD?

More . . .

1. What is attention deficit hyperactivity disorder (ADHD)?

Attention deficit hyperactivity disorder (ADHD) is a disorder in which a child displays hyperactive, impulsive, and/or inattentive behavior that is age-inappropriate. ADHD is a result of an atypical chemical balance in the brain, which means that ADHD is a physical problem, not an emotional problem. Outside factors, such as poor parenting, a chaotic home situation, divorce, or school stresses may affect how the symptoms come to light, but they do not cause ADHD. In order to diagnose ADHD (according to the *Diagnostic and Statistical Manual of Mental Disorders,* Fourth Edition, Text Revision [DSM-IV-TR]), problems of inattention and/or hyperactivity and impulsivity must interfere with a child's functioning in at least two settings (home, school, or social situations). In addition, the guidelines state that at least some symptoms must have been present before the age of 7 years.

ADHD is a result of an atypical chemical balance in the brain, which means that ADHD is a physical problem, not an emotional problem.

2. How common is ADHD?

ADHD is quite common; it is conservatively estimated to affect 3% to 5% of school-age children. Some reports suggest that as many as 4% to 8% or even an amazing 10% to 18% of children have ADHD. Thus, somewhere between 2 and 13 million American children have ADHD. Put another way, on the average, at least one child in every classroom has ADHD. ADHD results in millions of physician visits per year.

Approximately 60% of children with ADHD have symptoms that persist into adulthood. This means that close to 8 million adults (about 4% of the U.S. adult population) have ADHD. However, as ADHD is a behavioral disorder still lacking a specific biological marker, estimates of its frequency can be affected by a number of factors.

The method for making the diagnosis most certainly affects the estimated frequency. The current DSM-IV-TR standards, which allow both hyperactive–impulsive and inattentive subtypes, have resulted in higher rates of diagnosis than previous DSM standards, which placed a higher emphasis on hyperactivity as a diagnostic criterion. In other words, the frequency of the diagnosis increases when hyperactivity is not regarded as a necessary characteristic for ADHD diagnosis. The looser the requirements are, the greater the number of individuals included under the diagnostic umbrella.

The estimated frequency of ADHD also depends on who provides the information to make the diagnosis: parent, teacher, child, or physician. All have their own agendas to report. Teachers are seeing children through the lens of the classroom, where there are specific academic and behavioral expectations. In a class full of children, disruption by a single student can have a ripple effect. On the other hand, in a large class full of children, teachers may not notice the quietly inattentive child. Children may be less aware of their own symptoms. Adolescents, in particular, are notorious for underreporting and minimizing their symptoms. Parents view their children's behavior from the perspective of day-in, day-out living. Their perspective is intensive as well as long-term. On the one hand, they may minimize symptoms that they have been living with for years. On the other hand, the behavior seen under the intensive lens of daily living may make them keenly aware of things that go unnoticed by others. Physicians see children in a rather artificial setting, where the child is the focus of attention and may be on his or her best behavior. Conversely, some children are stressed by a visit to the doctor and will immediately demonstrate ADHD-like signs by wandering around the office, touching and picking up everything in sight.

The problem of varying perspectives is highlighted in one study that asked parents, teachers, and physicians to rate children with school problems as having or not having ADHD. Results indicated that approximately 10% were rated a unanimous "yes" and 30% a unanimous "no." However, parents, teachers, and physicians disagreed on the diagnosis of almost two-thirds of the children.

Studies using quantitative questionnaires to assess the level of agreement between parents, teachers, and children demonstrate more consistency among raters, but the specific questionnaire used affects the level of agreement. Some of the shorter questionnaires tend to diagnose ADHD less frequently because they emphasize hyperactivity and, subsequently, miss the inattentive children. Longer questionnaires, which consider multiple situations in which attention is required, yield greater agreement among raters and are probably more reliable diagnostic tools.

Younger children tend to have more classic symptoms and more hyperactivity.

The child's age at evaluation also makes a difference. Younger children tend to have more classic symptoms and more hyperactivity. Thus, the diagnosis is more likely to be made in these younger children than in older inattentive, nonhyperactive children.

ADHD seems to occur with differing frequency in different cultures. For example, ADHD appears to be more common in the United States than in Britain. A large British national study found the prevalence of hyperkinetic disorder (the British term for hyperactivity) to be only 1.4%. In Japan, a study that based diagnosis on an older version of the DSM (which places a greater emphasis on hyperactivity for diagnosis) determined that 8% of children in the general population met the standards for ADHD. The frequency of ADHD in two South American countries, Colombia and Venezuela, ranged from 7% to 11%. Studies coming out of Germany suggest a frequency of approximately 16%. The differences could be a reflection of different thresholds for diagnosis among different cultures or different diagnostic criteria (or both). For example, in Britain, hyperactivity appears to be a more important symptom for diagnosis than in the United States. The variation in frequency could also be a reflection of differing **gene pools** in these countries, with more ADHD genes in one population than in another.

Hyperkinetic

The British term for hyperactivity.

Gene pool

Genes for different disorders that are more or less common in particular populations.

3. Do different types of ADHD exist?

Yes. The DSM-IV-TR identifies three subtypes of ADHD (**Table 1**). Some children have symptoms that suggest a mainly hyperactive–impulsive type. To meet criteria for this subtype, a child must exhibit six or more symptoms (including restlessness, frequent interrupting, or talking excessively; see **Table 2** for the list of core symptoms). The second subtype emphasizes inattention. To have a diagnosis of this subtype of ADHD, a child must have difficulty following directions, fail to pay close attention to details, be forgetful in daily activities, or become easily distracted. In the third subtype, the combined type, a child must display six or more symptoms of both inattention and of hyperactivity–impulsivity.

Table 1   DSM-IV-TR Subtypes of ADHD

ADHD Subtype	How Subtype Is Determined
1. Predominantly inattentive type	Six or more symptoms of "inattention"
2. Predominantly hyperactive–impulsive type	Six or more symptoms of "hyperactivity–impulsivity"
3. Combined type	Six or more symptoms of inattention and six or more symptoms of hyperactivity–impulsivity

Definition: Patient has experienced symptoms and has been impaired for 6 months or greater.

Reprinted with permission from the *Diagnostic and Statistical Manual of Mental Disorders,* Fourth Edition, Text Revision. Copyright 2000 & DSM III American Psychiatric Association.

4. At what age does ADHD most often surface?

The disorder affects individuals of all ages. Of the millions of visits for ADHD to community physicians, about 5% are preschoolers, approximately 66% were elementary school-age, 20% were teenagers, and 15% were adults. ADHD is, however, most often diagnosed in elementary school-age children. Some children are diagnosed later during their junior high school and high school years. It also is not unusual for individuals to receive their first diagnosis of ADHD as adults. Interestingly, many parents first recognize that they have ADHD when it is diagnosed in their child. As this disorder was not diagnosed very frequently years ago, many individuals went through their school years with undiagnosed ADHD. Subsequently, when parents see their children experiencing similar difficulties, they remember their own history, are able to relate, and confirm their own undiagnosed disorder.

ADHD can be diagnosed in preschoolers. Indeed, the peak age of onset, which is different from the age at

Table 2   DSM-IV-TR Core Symptoms of ADHD in Children

Hyperactivity–Impulsivity

- Often fails to pay attention to details or makes careless mistakes in schoolwork, work, or other activities
- Often has difficulty in sustaining attention in tasks or play
- Often does not listen when spoken to directly
- Often does not follow through on instructions and fails to finish a project, etc.
- Often has difficulty in organizing tasks and activities
- Often avoids, dislikes, or is reluctant to engage in tasks that require sustained mental effort
- Often loses things necessary for tasks or activities
- Is often distracted by extraneous stimuli
- Is often forgetful in daily activities

Hyperactivity

- Often fidgets with hands or feet or squirms in seat
- Often leaves seat in classroom or in other situations in which it is inappropriate; in adults or adolescents, may be limited to subjective feelings of restlessness
- Often runs or climbs excessively in situations in which it is inappropriate; in adolescents or adults, may be limited to subjective feelings of restlessness
- Often has difficulty in playing or engaging in leisure activities quietly
- Is often "on the go" or acts as if "driven by a motor"
- Often talks excessively

Impulsivity

- Often blurts out answers before questions have been completed
- Often has difficulty in awaiting turn
- Often interrupts or intrudes on others
- Some hyperactive–impulsive or inattentive symptoms that caused impairment present before age 7
- Some impairment from the symptoms present in two or more settings (school, work, home)
- Clear evidence of significant impairment in social, academic, or occupational functioning
- Symptoms not accounted for by another disorder and do not occur exclusively during another disorder

Reprinted with permission from the *Diagnostic and Statistical Manual of Mental Disorders*, Fourth Edition, Text Revision. Copyright 2000 & DSM III American Psychiatric Association.

The Basics

diagnosis, may be between ages 3 and 4. Not surprisingly, severity affects the age at which ADHD is first noticed, with those more severely affected presenting at a younger age.

5. Do children outgrow ADHD?

Many children do outgrow ADHD. However, the latest data suggest that 50% to 70% of children continue to have some symptoms of ADHD in adolescence, and as many as 50% have persistent ADHD in adulthood. However, even in persistent cases, the number of symptoms decrease during adolescence and usually decrease further in adulthood. The types of symptoms also change. Hyperactivity and impulsivity tend to disappear, although adults with ADHD will often comment on their mental as opposed to physical restlessness. From a biological vantage point, the reduction of symptoms probably reflects brain maturation that continues through adolescence and beyond.

6. What parts of the brain are affected in ADHD?

In studies of ADHD children, the structures that most often have been found to play a role are the **frontal lobes**, the **striatum** (particularly the **caudate**), and the connection between these structures, which is called the **frontostriatal circuitry**. More recently, the **cerebellum** has also been found to play a role in ADHD (**Figure 1**).

If you are not a neurologist, that explanation probably does not mean much, so here is a quick lesson in brain anatomy and function. Your brain is made up of four lobes: frontal, parietal, temporal, and occipital. By and large, the frontal lobes control executive functioning

Even in persistent cases, the number of symptoms decrease during adolescence and usually decrease further in adulthood.

Frontal lobes

Front section of the brain that controls planning, organizing, starting, persisting, shifting, and inhibiting impulsive behaviors.

Striatum

Part of the basal ganglia, which consists of several interconnected regions/nuclei deep within the brain, specifically the caudate and putamen.

Caudate

Nucleus within the basal ganglia that appears to be most involved in ADHD. It is rich in dopamine and about 5% smaller in children with ADHD.

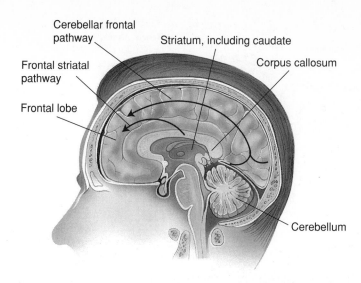

Cerebellar frontal pathway

Striatum, including caudate

Frontal striatal pathway

Corpus callosum

Frontal lobe

Cerebellum

Figure 1   The frontal lobes, the striatum, the cerebellum, and the connections between them are the areas of the brain that are crucial for attention.

The Basics

Frontostriatal circuitry

The connections between the frontal lobes of the brain and the basal ganglia that is located deeper within the brain.

Cerebellum

A brain structure in the hindbrain that is primarily involved in balance and coordination. Its role in cognitive and behavior disorders, including ADHD, has been recently discovered.

(e.g., planning, organizing, starting, persisting, shifting, and inhibiting impulsive behaviors). The **parietal lobes** control sensory functions and spatial skills (especially the right parietal lobe). The **temporal lobes** control language comprehension and memory, and the **occipital lobes** control vision. The left frontal lobe has the bigger effect on language-related executive functions, and the right frontal lobe has more of an influence on spatial executive function (**Figure 2**).

The striatum is made up of a number of structures deep within the brain, the caudate being the most active in ADHD. In healthy individuals, the striatum is rich in dopamine. Some structures in the striatum play a significant role in motor function. Parts of the striatum are low in dopamine in such movement disorders as Parkinson's disease, leading to tremors and very slow movements. Parts of the striatum have also been found to be involved in tic disorders (discussed in Question 37).

Parietal lobes

Midsection of the brain that controls sensory functions and also serves to integrate several brain functions simultaneously, such as seeing and hearing.

Temporal lobes

Lower section of the brain that controls memory and language comprehension.

Occipital lobes

Rear section of the brain that controls vision.

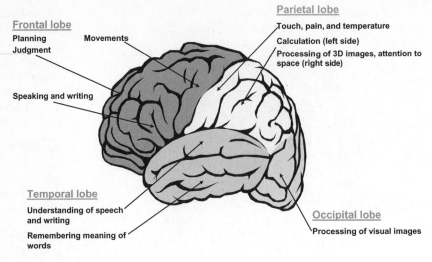

Figure 2 Localization of various functions in the human brain.

Neurotransmitters

Chemical messengers that allow neurons to communicate with one another by transferring information from one brain cell to another. Dopamine, norepinephrine, and serotonin are neurotransmitters implicated in ADHD.

Synapse

Specialized site between two neurons (brain cells) where neurotransmitters can pass from one cell to the next.

Neurons

Brain cells that can both send and receive information from other brain cells.

The frontostriatal circuitry forms the connection between the frontal lobes and parts of the striatum. Brain cells connect these structures, and the connection is maintained by information passed between the cells via neurotransmitters.

Finally, the cerebellum is part of the hindbrain and has been thought to primarily handle coordination. However, recent studies suggest it plays an important role in cognitive functions, such as language and attention, as well as motor planning. Cerebellar striatal frontal circuitry may also play a role in ADHD.

7. Where in the brain do neurotransmitters have their effects?

Neurotransmitters are chemicals in your brain that pass along information from one cell to another. Neurotransmitters act in the **synapse**, the space between two brain cells (**neurons**). Neurotransmitters released

The Basics

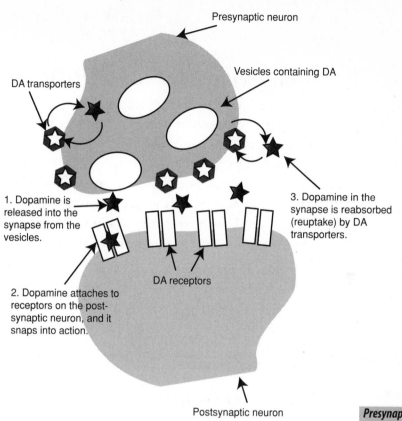

Presynaptic neuron

Vesicles containing DA

DA transporters

1. Dopamine is released into the synapse from the vesicles.

2. Dopamine attaches to receptors on the post-synaptic neuron, and it snaps into action.

3. Dopamine in the synapse is reabsorbed (reuptake) by DA transporters.

DA receptors

Postsynaptic neuron

Figure 3   Dopamine neurotransmission in ADHD.

by **presynaptic neurons** act on **receptors** on **postsyn-aptic neurons** (**Figure 3**). The amount of neurotrans-mitter in the synaptic space and the sensitivity of the postsynaptic cell receptors determine the neurotrans-mitter's effect on the postsynaptic brain cell.

There are many different neurotransmitters. Although dopamine is probably the neurotransmitter that is maximally involved in ADHD, norepinephrine and serotonin probably play lesser roles. The relative bal-ance among these neurotransmitters may be as impor-tant as their absolute amounts. Dopamine is the main

Presynaptic neuron

Sends the message by releasing a neurotransmitter.

Receptor

Places on neurons that bind neurotrans-mitters, or where medications act. Some medications can increase or decrease the number or sensitivity of receptors.

Postsynaptic neuron

Receives the message carried by the neuro-transmitter.

neurotransmitter in the striatum, while norepinephrine is the main neurotransmitter in the frontal lobe.

8. What genes are involved in ADHD?

You may be aware that many functions in our body, including production of hormones and other body and brain chemicals, are controlled by specific genes—the molecules of DNA that tell our cells how to develop and behave. You may not, however, have a clear idea of how this really works, and the fact is that scientists did not either until fairly recently. Mapping the human genome has helped determine some of the genes controlling specific functions, but many genes affect body systems in ways that scientists have yet to figure out. In some cases, multiple genes may be involved in complex interactions to cause an organ or a system to function properly (or improperly, as in the case of ADHD and many other disorders).

Genetic studies of ADHD have focused largely on genes involved in controlling the neurotransmitter dopamine (discussed in Question 51). This is logical because medications that increase dopamine are effective treatments for ADHD. Furthermore, brain-imaging studies have identified abnormalities in the dopamine-rich frontal and striatal regions in individuals with ADHD. In animal models used to investigate ADHD, "knock-out" mice—mice missing a gene important for increasing dopamine—are hyperactive and do not respond to stimulant treatment. Their dopamine can not be increased, and they remain hyperactive.

Currently the genes most likely to cause ADHD are thought to involve dopamine regulation. The **dopamine transporter (DAT)** gene is the prime candidate. This gene regulates the amount of dopamine in the synapse

Brain-imaging studies have identified abnormalities in the dopamine-rich frontal and striatal regions in individuals with ADHD.

Dopamine transporter (DAT)

An enzyme that transports dopamine back into the presynaptic neuron, lowering the level of dopamine in the synaptic space.

by determining how much dopamine is reabsorbed into the presynaptic neurons. In controls, the dopamine transporter keeps the level of dopamine in the synapse relatively high. In ADHD, the DAT "overfunctions" and lowers the level of synaptic dopamine. Stimulants inhibit DAT. As a result, more dopamine remains in the synapse (see Question 7). Other possible causal genes control postsynaptic dopamine receptors. They affect the sensitivity of the receptors to dopamine. It may take more dopamine to activate the postsynaptic receptors in children with ADHD.

So what does this knowledge mean for treating children with ADHD? First, it may help scientists design better medications for treating ADHD. They can target the cause of the neurotransmitter problem. Second, scientists can work toward treatments, called **gene therapy**, that correct the genetic abnormalities by replacing the abnormal gene. Gene treatment is currently being tried for a number of serious progressive neurological disorders.

Gene therapy

Treatments that correct the genetic abnormalities of conditions like ADHD.

9. Does having ADHD mean that something is fundamentally wrong with my child's brain?

ADHD is a biological, brain-based problem, but that's not the same as saying that something is wrong with your child's brain. There's a big difference between damage and dysfunction. Damage causes problems with the "hardware" or the basic brain structures. That's not what happens in ADHD. Although research data show that some brain structures, particularly the caudate, the **corpus callosum** (which allows the two hemispheres to "talk" to each other), and the cerebellum may be smaller in children with ADHD, but there is no indication that damage per se is present. In ADHD,

Corpus callosum

A structure that lies between the left and right hemisphere and is required for passing information between them. A role for the corpus callosum in ADHD has been recently hypothesized because it tends to be smaller than normal in children with ADHD by about 5%.

the primary problem is with the "software": the wiring or the connections in the brain. The problem with the connections most likely can be traced to atypical amounts of specific neurotransmitters, either individually or in relation to one another.

One recent imaging study showed that children with ADHD have relative cortical thinning in regions important for attention. Children with persistent ADHD had "fixed" thinning of areas of the frontal cortex, which may compromise the maturation of attentional systems. On the other hand, cortical thickness normalized in children who "outgrow" their ADHD.

10. Would I know any famous people who have or have had ADHD?

Most certainly ADHD has affected the lives of all kinds of people including authors, inventors, military leaders, statesmen, composers, athletes, and actors and actresses. The following list includes individuals who may or may not have had diagnosed ADHD but who most certainly exhibited behavior that indicates the possible presence of ADHD or other learning disabilities. For example, Danny Glover, Bill Cosby, Tom Cruise, Jim Carrey, Robin Williams, Nolan Ryan, Jason Kidd, and Magic Johnson are all individuals who have been described as having ADHD symptoms. Many very successful entrepreneurs, such as Walt Disney and Malcolm Forbes, have also proved that their ability to "think outside the box" was perhaps a more positive consequence of ADHD. In fact, many individuals who have excelled at multitasking may have been using features of their ADHD in a positive way; their difficulties in focusing on a single task improved their ability to handle many tasks at once.

PART TWO

Risk Factors, Symptoms, and Diagnosis

What causes ADHD?

If I have ADHD, will my child also have it?

Do the symptoms of ADHD change as children mature?

More . . .

RISK FACTORS

11. What causes ADHD?

Genetic proclivity

Likelihood that a disorder is passed from one generation to another by a gene or genes.

Heritability rate

Reflects the percentage of the cause of ADHD that is attributable to genetic as opposed to environmental factors. A heritability rate of 0.6 means that 60% of the cause of ADHD in an individual is genetic.

By far, the most common cause of ADHD is a **genetic proclivity** (i.e., ADHD is often inherited). Studies suggest that the heritability rate of ADHD ranges from 0.75 to 0.91. The **heritability rate** indicates the percentage of ADHD in an individual resulting from genetic rather than environmental factors. Thus, a heritability rate of 0.75 means that 75% of the cause of ADHD is genetic. However, ADHD can also be caused or exacerbated by other factors, such as preterm birth, anemia, medications for asthma, and other environmental factors. These factors are discussed later.

12. If I have ADHD, will my child also have it?

No, not necessarily, but the chance is definitely greater than if you did not have ADHD. For example, one-third of fathers with a history of ADHD in childhood have a child with ADHD. For mothers, the percentage is somewhat lower. Sometimes, it is a male relative in the mother's family who has ADHD. Mothers presumably have the ADHD gene, but they may exhibit few or no symptoms. Nonetheless, these mothers can pass the ADHD gene on to their children. We are still not sure why females are less likely to have ADHD symptoms, even when it is almost certain they have one of the ADHD genes. In one study of ADHD adults and controls, 43% of children with ADHD parents met criteria for a diagnosis of ADHD, compared to 2% of children in the control group of children who had parents without ADHD. If your first child has ADHD, the risk of your second child having ADHD is probably higher than in the general population. However, predicting

If your first child has ADHD, the risk of your second child having ADHD is probably higher than in the general population.

the severity of ADHD or the type of ADHD that might run in a family is not possible.

13. Do nongenetic risk factors for ADHD exist?

Results from a large national study performed in the 1960s indicated that a number of nongenetic factors can affect the risk of ADHD. The children evaluated in that study were followed from conception until 7 years of age. Risk factors for ADHD included a history of smoking, alcohol use, drug use or anemia during pregnancy, breech birth, chorioamnionitis (infection of the placenta) during labor, premature birth, and small head size at birth. A family history of mental retardation and low socioeconomic status also appeared to be risk factors. **Neurological** problems in the first month of life increase the risk of ADHD at age 7 years from 2% to 50%. In infancy, delayed development and increased activity predict ADHD at age 7 years. When a 4-year-old child has a small head size, astigmatism, or visual motor, fine motor, or gross motor deficits, the risk of ADHD is increased.

Psychosocial problems at home are also risk factors for ADHD. A Hawaiian study revealed a 200% to 400% increased risk of ADHD in children from families where there was a lot of conflict in the home. In a Swedish study, unsatisfactory family life was the largest risk factor for ADHD, overriding any other medical problems.

Having a risk factor or even several risk factors does not mean that ADHD is going to occur, but it makes ADHD more likely than in someone who has no risk factors. The various risk factors predispose a child to ADHD to different degrees.

Neurological
Refers to functions controlled by the brain.

Psychosocial
The impact of social situations and mental health upon each other.

14. Was my child born with ADHD, or did it "develop?"

In most cases, to the extent that ADHD is a genetic disorder, your child was born with ADHD. In other words, the genes that contribute to the disorder were present at birth. Some children born with the genes for the disorder do not develop ADHD symptoms at all; some have such slight difficulties with attention that it goes undetected throughout their lives. Nevertheless, the signs can appear and change over time, depending on a variety of circumstances. Environmental factors play a role even when the main cause is genetic. A child with a mild disorder can subsequently manifest extreme inattention or hyperactive behavior in the presence of certain environmental factors, such as parental abuse or neglect, poor living conditions, or other circumstances that stress children emotionally. If ADHD symptoms develop "suddenly," it is likely that the disorder was present but hidden, only appearing when an environmental factor came into play.

15. My child with ADHD can sit and watch TV for hours, but I have heard that watching television can cause ADHD. Is this true?

Researchers have recently reported that for every hour a day preschoolers watch television, their risk of developing ADHD increases by about 10%. These new findings are consistent with previous research showing that television can shorten attention spans. Researchers have speculated that TV might actually overstimulate and permanently "rewire" the developing brain.

The newest study on TV watching assessed more than 1000 children. Parents were questioned about the

Researchers have recently reported that for every hour a day preschoolers watch television, their risk of developing ADHD increases by about 10%.

children's TV watching habits at 1 and 3 years of age. They rated their children's behavior at age 7 years on a scale commonly used to diagnose ADHD. About 10% met criteria for a diagnosis of ADHD, about the same frequency as is usually found in 7-year-olds. But the 37% of 1-year-olds who watched 1 to 2 hours daily had a 10% to 20% increased risk of attention problems; the 14% who watched 3 to 4 hours daily had a 30% to 40% increased risk compared with children who watched no TV. Among 3-year-olds, only 7% watched no TV, 44% watched 1 to 2 hours daily, 27% watched 3 to 4 hours daily, almost 11% watched 5 to 6 hours daily, and about 10% watched 7 or more hours daily. These children too were at increased risk for ADHD, and the risk was proportionate to how much TV they watched. Although the research has been done on TV watching, the effects of any repetitive non-educational activity or electronic device, such as playing video games, may be the same.

The TV research is compelling enough that the American Academy of Pediatrics recommends that parents do not permit children under 2 years of age to watch television because of concerns that it affects early brain growth and the development of social, emotional, and **cognitive skills**. And there are many other reasons that children should not watch television. For example, TV watching has been associated with obesity and aggressiveness. So, even if it is one of the places your ADHD child will sit quietly, it is best to limit TV watching. You need to be creative about finding other things your child would like to do. Reading to your child or encouraging your child to read alone, even if he is reading sports magazines or comic books, is a better alternative.

Cognitive skills

Pertaining to cognition, the process of knowing and, more precisely, the process of being aware, knowing, thinking, learning, and judging.

16. What other environmental factors may cause ADHD?

Although environmental factors are most certainly not the main elements leading to ADHD, evidence suggests that exposures to various agents, such as drugs, chemicals, or illnesses, may increase the risk of ADHD. For example, iron-deficiency anemia (discussed in Question 19) and thyroid disorders can cause problems with attention span. Exposure to such substances as lead and mercury may also increase the chances of a child having ADHD.

17. Can a significant head injury or a minor concussion cause ADHD?

Behavior problems from significant traumatic brain injury include irritability, fatigue, impulsiveness, decreased anger control, disinhibition, decreased motivation, decreased frustration tolerance, decreased initiative, aggressiveness, decreased attention, and hypo- or hyperactivity. This is due at least in part to the fact that a closed-head injury is likely to damage the frontal lobes of the brain. A physician must carefully and indefinitely monitor the classroom attention of a child who has sustained a significant head injury. In contrast, concussions, which are associated with only a brief loss of consciousness, are considered very minor head injuries. Nonetheless, children may have trouble concentrating and focusing for several weeks after a concussion. The effects are transient, but can temporarily affect school performance. Paying attention to the problem will minimize it.

18. Are children born prematurely at increased risk for ADHD?

The frequency of ADHD in children born prematurely is fairly high.

The frequency of ADHD in children born prematurely is fairly high. One study compared children who had been born prematurely with children who were from the same social class but had been born at full-term. When the children were evaluated at age 7 years, approximately 20% of those in the premature group had ADHD as compared to about 10% of the other group. Many of the premature children who had ADHD also had additional cognitive, neurological, or academic disabilities (e.g., **dyslexia** and developmental language disorders).

Dyslexia

A specific reading disability due to a defect in the brain's processing of graphic symbols.

The rapid advances in medical technology have greatly increased the number of children who survive premature birth. However, as more premature babies survive, there is growing evidence that suggests that there are long term repercussions: many of these children—especially the very small ones—develop major neurological problems. These children appear to be at special risk for ADHD because their frontostriatal circuitry is particularly vulnerable to injury owing to its immaturity at the time of birth. It is wise to carefully monitor children who are born premature.

19. My child with iron-deficiency anemia is hyperactive rather than tired. Is that common?

Anemia, although commonly thought to decrease energy, can be a cause of inattention and hyperactivity during early childhood. Pediatricians routinely monitor for anemia, which is most often caused by iron deficiency. Iron replacement corrects both the anemia and the inattention and hyperactivity fairly quickly.

20. Could the many ear infections my child had as a toddler be the cause of his ADHD?

Some studies, although not all, have found that children with a history of frequent bilateral ear infections had lower language and speech scores, lower reading scores, and more behavior and attention problems during elementary school. Investigators have suggested that children who suffer from intermittent hearing impairments from ear infections do not get enough "practice" in paying attention. This does not mean that your child will have problems in these areas if he has frequent ear infections, but parents and teachers do need to be vigilant about this problem. It is very unlikely that ADHD is caused by ear infections.

SYMPTOMS

21. At what age might I begin to worry about whether my child has ADHD? Can ADHD be diagnosed in a preschooler?

ADHD can be diagnosed in a child as young as 3 years of age.

ADHD can be diagnosed in a child as young as 3 years of age. Signs of ADHD in preschoolers may include a noticeably high activity level, inability to persist with tasks, problems in following group instructions, poor behavior modulation, difficulties with social interactions, unending curiosity, excessive aggression or destructive play, silliness, bossiness, and impulsivity. Preschoolers with ADHD may have sleep problems, such as restless or decreased sleep. In addition, argumentative behavior and temper tantrums may be more common in preschoolers with ADHD. These children may also be quite immature, frequently demonstrating off-task or inappropriate behaviors. All of this can contribute to conflicts within the family, ranging from battles with siblings and parents to difficulties in keeping baby-sitters.

22. Do the symptoms of ADHD change as children mature?

Yes. Although some symptoms persist, many symptoms of ADHD change with development. For example, hyperactivity diminishes in some children after elementary school. Many people think that the hormonal changes of puberty are responsible for this, although we do not understand the mechanism. Older children may have either outgrown their hyperactivity or found ways in which to channel it. A sense of inner restlessness may replace the hyperactivity. In the preteen and adolescent years, poor grades, inability to sustain attention, difficulties in maintaining social relationships, disorganization, and risk-taking behavior may surface as primary symptoms. At school, ADHD may show up more as written work becomes increasingly complex and a teenager is required to plan ahead for long-term assignments. Socially, the range of accepted behavior in many ways is narrowed by the unwritten rules of a teenager's peer group. The difficulties with emotional self-control and interpersonal communication common in ADHD makes these teenagers appear more immature and clumsy among their peers. Their impulsivity may cause them to blurt out answers inappropriately or to interrupt conversations. They can become disruptive in the classroom or even be perceived as the "class clown." This can result in peer rejection and subsequent distress in ADHD children.

23. Are there other signs of ADHD besides the ones traditionally used to establish the diagnosis?

ADHD can show up in children in many ways besides those defined by established criteria in DSM-IV-TR. Social-skill issues may be the presenting symptoms at home and at school. Children may display isolated aggressive behavior in preschool and early elementary school, because of their impulsivity and poor attention to verbal and visual cues. Because their disruptive behavior often results in conflicts with peers, siblings, and authority figures, such children stand out from their classmates. Consequently, they tend to be rejected by their peers. Children with ADHD may also be quite messy and disorganized. Parents frequently describe bedrooms in complete disarray, backpacks with papers falling out, and poor eating habits. General academic difficulties are also common. Children forget their assignments, do not appear to be listening in class, and get poor grades. In addition, they may have what are usually called executive functioning problems: difficulties with planning, starting tasks, shifting from one activity to another, controlling responses, and staying interested and motivated.

24. Do ADHD symptoms in late adolescence put my child at risk for other kinds of problems?

The persistence of ADHD symptoms into adolescence is associated with more academic, behavioral, and social problems. Research indicates that adults with continuing symptoms complete less formal schooling, are employed at the usual rates but have lower-status jobs, and have higher rates of personality disorders. The frequency of **substance abuse** is higher among adolescents and young adults with continuing ADHD. Coexisting conduct and antisocial personality disorders further increase the risk of substance abuse.

Recent research comparing children who outgrow ADHD to those who remain symptomatic suggests that those with persisting ADHD are more likely to develop other associated illnesses (e.g., conduct and oppositional disorders), which can become increasingly prominent and problematic for these adolescents and young adults. The risk-taking and rule-breaking behavior can also significantly worsen parent–child conflicts.

Research indicates that adults with continuing symptoms complete less formal schooling, are employed at the usual rates but have lower-status jobs, and have higher rates of personality disorders.

Substance abuse

Self-administration of any drug in a culturally disapproved manner that has adverse consequences.

Among children whose symptoms decrease during adolescence, the outcome is similar to that of non-ADHD individuals regarding occupational achievement, social functioning, and drug and alcohol use, although not academic achievement. Academic issues may remain an affected area even if ADHD disappears.

25. Does everyone with attention problems or hyperactivity have ADHD?

No. There are many potential causes for behaviors similar to that seen in ADHD. Children with language disorders who have difficulty understanding and/or expressing themselves can appear inattentive. Their experience may be similar to listening to a foreign language in which words are picked up only here and there. Because they do not always understand what a teacher is saying, such children lose their focus. Consequently, deciding whether a child with language problems also has ADHD can sometimes be difficult. Some children with specific medical problems may also appear to be inattentive. For example, thyroid problems can cause attention difficulties. On the one hand, too little thyroid hormone may cause a child to become inattentive; on the other, too much thyroid hormone may cause hyperactivity. Children with seizures may appear inattentive, but this usually occurs irregularly and only when the seizures are occurring. Children with sleep problems may also appear inattentive because they are so tired during the day. A child with any one of a variety of emotional difficulties may also appear unable to concentrate or may become hyperactive. Children with anxiety or depression sometimes appear preoccupied or distracted. In addition, unlike adults, depressed children may become quite agitated or restless, which can be mistaken for hyperactivity.

Obsessive-compulsive disorder (OCD)

A disorder in which individuals experience obsessions and/or compulsions.

As a rule, children with ADHD tend to be distracted by outside stimuli. In contrast, a child with **obsessive-compulsive disorder** or a psychotic illness, for example, may be distracted by internal events, recurring thoughts, and excessive worry. However, a casual observer cannot always tell the difference by the child's behavior, so it is difficult to correctly identify the source of the problem without careful assessment.

Inattentiveness and hyperactivity also can be side effects of medications. This is particularly common with some of the medications used for treating asthma, particularly theophylline and steroids. Antiseizure medicines can also interfere with attention.

Attention problems and hyperactivity are not automatically signs of ADHD, so you should not assume your child has ADHD because you see these behaviors.

In short, attention problems and hyperactivity are not automatically signs of ADHD, so you should not assume your child has ADHD because you see these behaviors. The child should be assessed by a professional trained to recognize the origins of behavioral problems so that the real cause or causes can be determined.

26. Does gender have an effect on ADHD in children?

Most studies indicate that more boys than girls have ADHD. The ratio is probably 2–3:1 in school-age children. One study that researched the frequency of ADHD in school-aged children in the United States found the rate in boys was 9% compared to a rate of 3% in girls. Age seems to have an effect on the gender ratio. The male:female ratio drops in adolescence toward 1:1. In fact, some adult studies even suggest that women have ADHD more often than men. As hyperactivity lessens, the inattentive form of ADHD more commonly seen in girls may persist and equalize the ratio.

Bear in mind, however, that these study results are determined by the detection of ADHD. Gender ratios may be affected by referral practices. Among children referred to child psychiatrists or psychologists, the boy–girl ratio varies from 3:1 to 9:1, whereas in community surveys of school-age children, it is closer to 2:1. More severely or obviously affected children are probably referred to a specialist and are usually boys. It is possible, however, that ADHD goes undetected in girls more often than it does in boys. In this regard, it is important to note that boys and girls tend to have different types of ADHD. Boys more often have the hyperactive–impulsive type or the combined type, whereas girls more often have the inattentive type. Some people suggest that this difference affects the frequency with which ADHD is picked up. In other words, boys could receive diagnoses more often because they are more vocal, their problematic behavior is more obvious, and they are more troublesome for their teachers and families. Although girls tend to be affected less often than are their male peers, some studies suggest that those with diagnosed ADHD tend to be less bright and have more academic difficulties than do boys with ADHD. It is possible that very bright girls simply compensate better and their ADHD goes undetected.

27. Often, when I say no, my child overreacts and is defiant or hostile. Is that common for a child with ADHD?

Not every ADHD child is defiant, hostile, or oppositional. However, some are. A certain amount of defiant and oppositional behavior is normal in children of all ages. Yet, it may be a more common or more prominent issue with ADHD children (discussed in Question 91). These children may interrupt and intrude as well as avoid tasks or directions. They may also deliberately annoy other people and blame others for something they themselves do. In fact, accepting responsibility for their behavior may be quite hard for them. However, you must distinguish their inattention and impulsivity from the disruptive behaviors in truly hostile children. Specific characteristics seen in a child with an **oppositional defiant disorder** include poor temper control, argumentativeness, spitefulness and vindictiveness ("getting even"), resentfulness and anger, and the tendency to rebel against or refuse adult requests. ADHD children can sometimes be defiant and hostile. But, when your ADHD child routinely becomes disruptive and argumentative, it's time for a professional consultation to determine whether your child has a comorbid disorder. In other words, such children can have two separate problems that occur at the same time.

Oppositional defiant disorder

A disorder characterized by negative, hostile, and defiant behavior that causes significant damage in social, academic, or occupational interactions.

DIAGNOSIS

28. What are the essential elements of a thorough evaluation to diagnose ADHD?

A thorough evaluation of ADHD requires the recording of a detailed history from parents, a discussion with or observation of the affected child, and some backup evidence from someone outside the home. A qualified doctor can accomplish this at an appointment with you and your child. Although the diagnosis will generally be apparent from a child's history, an interviewer most likely will ask you, your child, and your child's teachers to complete appropriate questionnaires.

A detailed history is essential to diagnosing ADHD. It should include information about your child's birth; illnesses; early language and motor milestones; infant, toddler, and preschool years; educational progress and motivation; homework habits; social interactions and interests; and hobbies and extracurricular activities. A family medical and social history is also important. A detailed history will often include anecdotes that give the doctor a more complete picture of your child's past and present.

The diagnosis of ADHD requires that the child have symptoms that interfere in at least two settings. By definition, outside sources are required. Although getting a description directly from a teacher—by questionnaire or in person—is useful, parents' description of what they have been told about classroom behavior often suffices. Sometimes, teacher questionnaires are useful not only for diagnosis, but to show parents how a teacher rates their child's attention and behavior in a quantitative, rather than a qualitative or descriptive way (such as they would hear at a parent–teacher conference).

The diagnosis of ADHD requires that the child have symptoms that interfere in at least two settings. By definition, outside sources are required.

A doctor will also try to obtain a complete "picture" of your child. This may involve performing a physical examination, asking questions about school and outside interests, or asking your child to do some simple tasks (e.g., walking on toes and heels or drawing a picture). The objective is to develop an accurate sense of your child for diagnostic purposes.

29. Whom do I consult to get a proper diagnosis of ADHD?

A number of different kinds of doctors can diagnose ADHD. Which type you choose to examine your child depends in part on your access to subspecialists and in part on the degree of ADHD and the presence of accompanying disorders. A regular pediatrician or a developmental pediatrician (a pediatrician who specializes in learning issues) can generally manage a child with relatively mild ADHD. Both neurologists and psychiatrists diagnose and treat children with ADHD. Often, they see children whose ADHD is complicated by other medical or psychiatric problems. Pediatricians may refer a patient to either a neurologist or a psychiatrist when the diagnosis is unclear or when they feel that adequately managing an affected child is becoming difficult. A psychiatrist might be a particularly good option for a child with comorbid problems involving oppositional behavior, anxiety, or mood. Conversely, a neurologist might be the right choice for a child with comorbid **tics**, **Tourette's syndrome**, or a specific neurological problem (e.g., seizures).

Although psychologists can not prescribe medication, they can diagnose and treat problems associated with ADHD. However, several types of psychologists are available, and their methods of assessment will differ. Clinical psychologists may use techniques similar to those of a psychiatrist. They will interview parents and child, gaining both historical and current information about developmental, academic, social, and emotional issues and other aspects of the child's behavior. Other psychologists, usually educational psychologists or neuropsychologists, will use more quantitative measurements to make a diagnosis. Besides following the more typical interview procedures, these clinicians will perform several hours of testing to arrive at a diagnosis. Most certainly, significant school difficulties or outstanding social and emotional issues are symptoms that may warrant a more complete assessment by a psychologist, either through the board of education or on a private basis. In this way, a fuller picture of a child's particular strengths and weaknesses can be obtained.

Tics

Involuntary muscle movements or twitches.

Tourette's syndrome

A disorder characterized by numerous motor and vocal tics. To be diagnosed with Tourette's, tics must be present for at least 1 year.

30. I took my child to a doctor who made the diagnosis in 30 minutes. Can doctors really make a diagnosis of ADHD that quickly?

Yes. Although parents may have difficulty understanding this, professionals may be able to make the diagnosis of ADHD quite quickly. First, as qualified professionals, they see many children with the same set of critical characteristics. Similar to diagnosing a medical condition, such as diabetes, a personal history in combination with symptoms may quickly point to the right diagnosis. In fact, a child's personal history alone is often the most important part of the diagnosis. In addition, if you and your child have provided the doctor with completed questionnaires that point out problems with inattention, hyperactivity, or impulsivity, the diagnosis is often immediately apparent. Very often the history is confirmed by a child's unruly behavior in the office: however, the key element of the diagnosis is the history, not the inappropriate office behavior.

Amy's comment[1]:

I was struck by how quickly Zachary was diagnosed. However, it didn't make me question the diagnosis; it made me realize that to some extent I was in denial, and it also validated my own feelings and suspicions about his behavior.

Although a doctor can come to an opinion rapidly, it doesn't mean that a parent will be comfortable with a diagnosis that is made so quickly and easily. Parents in such a situation naturally will question doctors about why and how they made the diagnosis. In fact, you may want to think about and discuss the diagnosis for a few days. It might be

Very often the history is confirmed by a child's unruly behavior in the office; however, the key element of the diagnosis is the history, not the inappropriate office behavior.

---

[1]Parental comments included in this book are inserted under invented names to protect the identity of the patients.

helpful to call the doctor back to discuss your questions. It is always a good idea to write your questions down so that you have them when you make your phone call. In the end, you and your child will choose what diagnosis you accept and what treatment options you pursue. If you are uncomfortable with the physician's qualifications or manner, you should seek a second opinion from another physician. Be aware, however, that insurance doesn't always cover second opinions.

31. Can medical tests reliably determine whether my child has ADHD?

Electroencephalo-gram (EEG)

A test that measures brain electrical activity.

Magnetic resonance imaging (MRI)

A technique that creates three-dimensional images of brain structures using strong magnetic fields.

functional Magnetic resonance imaging (fMRI)

MRI of the brain done while an activity is being performed that is formatted in a way to show where that activity is happening. For example, an fMRI done during an executive function task will show maximal activity in the frontal lobe.

No, ADHD is determined by a clinical diagnosis based on interviews and a child's personal history from teachers, parents, and others who are involved with the child on a day-to-day basis. Research studies using an **electroencephalogram (EEG)** to measure brain electrical activity, **magnetic resonance imaging (MRI)** to assess brain structure, and **functional magnetic resonance imaging (fMRI)** to measure where things happen in the brain have demonstrated some minor differences between the brains of ADHD children and those without ADHD (Question 9). These differences are found in brain regions we think are important for attention. However, EEG, MRI, and fMRI can not be used to make a diagnosis at this time. The findings are not consistent enough to be useful. Perhaps in the future this will change. In addition, even though research studies suggest neurotransmitter and neuroreceptor differences between children with and without ADHD, no blood tests are available to use to make the diagnosis. Although it is possible that researchers will develop some diagnostic laboratory test that can simplify diagnosis, it is unlikely to happen in the near future. Furthermore, even when we document the gene(s) causing ADHD, having the gene will not necessarily mean having ADHD. The human nervous system is just too complex for a simple one-to-one effect. Ultimately, a diagnosis of ADHD relies on the experience and judgment of the physician who examines the child, not medical tests or scans.

32. Is a psychoeducational or neuropsychological assessment really necessary?

Professionals can make a diagnosis of ADHD without testing. In other words, they can determine that a child has ADHD without administering a battery of educational, psychological, or neuropsychological tests. However, a thorough assessment of your child's strengths and weaknesses is an important tool to confirm diagnosis, to flesh out the consequences of difficulties with attention, and to determine the presence of comorbid disorders, such as learning disabilities or emotional problems.

Finishing a complete psychoeducational or **neuropsychological assessment** can take 7 to 10 hours. With a young child, that generally requires three to four sessions. Sometimes adolescents can work longer and complete the tests in one or two lengthy sittings. However, there is something to be said for seeing a student on multiple occasions when differences in their day-to-day concentration and mood may be apparent.

Whether your child has a psychoeducational or a neuropsychological assessment generally depends on whom you choose to perform the evaluation. Differences in the assessment basically involve differences in the evaluator's education and orientation. Any evaluation should look at different aspects of your child's functioning. Most certainly, the examiner should use a measure of

They can determine that a child has ADHD without administering a battery of educational, psychological, or neuropsychological tests.

Neuropsychological assessment

A series of tests used to examine the behavioral expression of brain function.

intellectual functioning and tests of academic achievement that cover the basics: reading, writing, and arithmetic. Other tests should measure your child's capacity to process material and use memory, language, visual-spatial, and sensory-motor skills. In addition, it is critical to have an examination of your child's executive functioning abilities. Executive functioning ability is a neuropsychological term that refers to skills controlled by the frontal lobe of the brain. Fundamentally, executive functioning skills tap your child's ability to "initiate, shift, sustain, and inhibit." Assessment of these skills includes an examination of the child's planning and organization, cognitive flexibility, sustained attention, and censoring abilities. Your child needs executive skills to be successful at academic tasks, to interact socially, and to adjust to changes in daily routine.

A thorough evaluation should also include some measures of social and emotional functioning.

A thorough evaluation should also include some measures of social and emotional functioning. Both self-report and projective measures can be used to assess those areas. A self-report questionnaire can focus on a particular area of functioning, such as anxiety or social skills. A thorough assessment also might require a much longer list of behaviors to be endorsed or rated and then analyzed to determine children's own outlook on their academic, emotional, and social functioning. Projective testing, conversely, involves the use of measures that encourage children to "project" their feelings and attitudes on a relatively neutral stimulus. For example, children tell a story about a picture or explain what they see in an inkblot. This is an excellent way for the examiner to obtain a better picture of children's underlying emotional status.

A psychologist will then compile and analyze data from all these sources, interpret the results, come to conclusions, and share them with the parents during a feedback session. Experts also encourage adolescents to receive direct feedback from the psychologist, as such children are old enough to appreciate their own strengths and weaknesses and to understand the meanings of a diagnosis. Once they understand the implications of the disorder, teenagers can become active participants in the treatment process. In this way, the feedback is actually the first step in their learning how to take on the responsibilities of handling ADHD for themselves.

33. I hear that ADHD is becoming more frequent among school children. Is it being overdiagnosed?

ADHD diagnoses increased dramatically in the 1990s. Although this is true, it's probably due to factors other than an increasing number of children with ADHD. First, awareness of the disorder is greater among clinicians, teachers, and parents. Second, the measures for ADHD have changed over the years. When evidence of hyperactivity was no longer required for diagnosis, the frequency definitely increased. Third, some suggest that the increased frequency reflects some new "advantages" of having diagnosed ADHD. Changes to the Individuals with Disabilities Education Act (IDEA; see Question 83), which officially recognized ADHD as a disorder in 1991, meant that children with ADHD became entitled to special school accommodations. For example, teachers grant ADHD children extra time on tests, provide them with tutoring, give them less homework, or penalize them less for handing in late assignments. Furthermore, extended time for such tests as the SATs is no longer flagged. This means that colleges are sent SAT scores but are not notified that an adolescent received extra time. Some argue that these changes have caused parents to seek out or accept the diagnosis more readily in exchange for services for their children, resulting in the steep increase in the diagnosis of ADHD and the resultant prescription of stimulants to treat it.

34. Since diagnostic criteria indicate that symptoms of ADHD are supposed to be present by 7 years of age, how can a doctor now suggest for the first time that my 13-year-old seventh grader has ADHD?

During their elementary school years, some children, particularly intelligent ones, can compensate for their problems with inattention. In other words, the academic workload is so easy for them that they do not need to be very organized or attentive to perform well. Middle-school curriculum makes new demands on executive functions by stressing the need for organizing, working independently, and using working memory (juggling more than two ideas at the same time). Children may not begin to have difficulties until the increasing academic expectations of middle school require them to be more organized, change classes, plan ahead, attend for prolonged lengths of time, and do long-term projects. Also, the departmentalized experience of middle school requires that they have more than one teacher, which can tax the executive abilities of even non-ADHD children. Therefore, students must adjust to different teaching styles. Instead of having one teacher who is very involved with a classroom of students, children have multiple teachers who know less about them and may be less tolerant of their ADHD. Previously masked symptoms will become more apparent. Older children are also more articulate about their own distractibility and inattentiveness, reporting it more spontaneously to those who inquire about their symptoms.

35. Is a child with ADHD more susceptible to other disorders as well?

Although children with ADHD may simply have problems with attention and concentration, it is also true that several issue areas are commonly associated with ADHD. In fact, diagnosis can be complicated because children with ADHD so often have additional symptoms and difficulties. Some of these children may have what is termed **subclinical** forms of other disorders. This means that although they do not have enough characteristics of another disorder to meet criteria for diagnosis, they do have isolated and mild symptoms. However, many other children with ADHD do suffer from comorbid disorders. Describing a disorder with high **comorbidity** means that a child with one disorder has a high likelihood of having another disorder. For example, some children with ADHD have motor coordination difficulties, language disorders, and/or learning disabilities. Doctors and parents should also carefully watch children with ADHD for difficulties with mood and anxiety. In addition, such other disorders as Tourette's syndrome, obsessive-compulsive disorder, oppositional defiant disorder, and **conduct disorder** have been associated with ADHD.

Approximately 50% of children with ADHD have one or more comorbid psychiatric disorder. Psychiatric problems can make the treatment of ADHD more difficult, and can in and of itself seriously complicate a child's life. Medication, psychotherapy, and/or academic accommodations may be necessary.

Diagnosis can be complicated because children with ADHD so often have additional symptoms and difficulties.

Subclinical

A form of a disease with very mild symptoms, often barely noticeable. In inherited disorders, family members who must be affected based on the genetic pattern of the disease, but who do not appear to be obviously affected, are described as having subclinical symptoms.

Comorbidity

Presence of two or more disorders in the same individual.

Conduct disorder

A disorder in which there is an active transgression of societal rules.

36. My child is very clumsy and hates team sports. Is that a common problem in children with ADHD?

Yes, some ADHD children have difficulties with motor coordination. Trouble sticking to motor tasks is common, as are difficulties with inhibiting inappropriate motor responses. It is also worth noting that children with motor coordination difficulties tend to do better in individual sports. Swimming, tennis, golf, fencing, and track are good choices for the ADHD child. On the other hand, youngsters learn a great deal about social interaction, cooperation, and how to handle competition when they play team sports. A child with ADHD may have trouble at the beginning, but they may become great team players over time.

37. My child with ADHD bites his nails, chews on his clothing, and frequently blinks his eyes. Is that part of his ADHD, or does he have tics?

The reported frequency of ADHD in children with Tourette's ranges from to 20% to 90%.

The reported frequency of ADHD in children with Tourette's ranges from to 20% to 90%; that of Tourette's in ADHD children ranges from to 10% to 50%. Tourette's has even been dubbed "ADHD with tics." In some children ADHD is probably a manifestation of the Tourette's gene(s) as opposed to the ADHD gene(s). In other words, instead of or in addition to causing tics, the Tourette's gene(s) causes ADHD. The brain and neurotransmitter abnormalities found in Tourette's overlap those seen in ADHD (discussed in Questions 7 and 53). Specifically, abnormalities of the fronto-striatal system and of dopamine metabolism are found in both disorders.

Tics are repeated movements or sounds that are involuntary. At times a child can temporarily suppress them. Tics are not steady or constant; in fact, they come and go. Some tics can actually be very mild, even going unnoticed by anyone but a professional. Some motor tics are simple, such as blinking, shoulder shrugging, or facial grimacing. When you stop to think about it, nail biting and knuckle cracking are actually tics, but they're so common that we tend not to really categorize them as tics. We call them habits. Some motor tics are more complex, such as jumping. Some children also exhibit **vocal tics**, which range from throat clearing and coughing to cursing. Cursing, however, is very uncommon.

Vocal tics

Involuntary sounds like throat clearing, sniffing, or words.

Temporary motor tics, which last from weeks to months, are rather common in school-age children and are conservatively reported to occur in 1 of 100 boys and in 1 of 500 girls. Some studies report transient tics in as many as 20% of school-aged children. Tics generally start around 7 years of age, which is usually a few years later than the appearance of initial signs of ADHD. In most children, tics lessen substantially or disappear in adolescence.

Although minor childhood tic disorders may be fairly widespread, Tourette's is less common, although definitely not rare. The frequency of Tourette's is 0.1% to 0.3% in the general school population and as high as 10% in special education populations. Tourette's disorder is characterized by a number of motor tics and by one or more vocal tics. To be diagnosed with Tourette's, a child must have tics that are present for at least 1 year and vary in type and frequency over time. Tourette's can also lessen substantially or disappear in adolescence.

38. Is my ADHD child's anxiety about school due to poor academic performance, or can ADHD children have co-occurring anxiety disorder?

Studies have determined that anxiety disorders occur in as many as 25% of children with ADHD.

Anxiety disorders can occur in children who have ADHD. In fact, studies have determined that anxiety disorders occur in as many as 25% of children with ADHD. Anxiety is a normal emotion for everyone. However, children with a true anxiety disorder experience these feelings more often, more easily, and more intensely than others. These children feel tension, worry, or uneasiness even when they have nothing to fear.

DSM-IV-TR describes several types of anxiety disorders. For example, children with separation-anxiety disorder have an extreme fear of being away from home or separated from their routine caretaker. Children with generalized-anxiety disorder are overanxious and worry about everything. Children with social phobia are painfully shy and uncomfortable in routine social situations. Panic disorder, agoraphobia (fear of the outdoors), specific phobia, and obsessive-compulsive disorder are also types of anxiety disorder. Note that while anxiety disorders are relatively common, they are infrequently associated with serious limitations in functioning and often go unnoticed by families.

It is also possible that children with ADHD can become anxious as a result of their ADHD. In such cases, they become more tense or nervous about peer relationships, academic performance, or meeting daily routines. In other words, the trouble in academic or psychosocial arenas that ADHD children face can cause them to become anxious. Most certainly, children with ADHD and anxiety—whether it is truly a comorbid anxiety disorder or a temporary problem stemming from their ADHD—may be at risk for school phobia or academic problems.

While quite uncommon, it should be noted that stimulants can exacerbate underlying anxiety disorders. If your child becomes more anxious when stimulants are started or the dose is increased, let your physician know.

39. How often do obsessive-compulsive disorder and ADHD co-occur?

Studies suggest an overlap of somewhere between 6% and 33% between obsessive-compulsive disorder and ADHD. As with anxiety, stimulant medications can on occasion exacerbate underlying OCD. However, more often the appearance of OCD in a child with ADHD is unrelated to medication.

Obsessive-compulsive disorder, as defined in the DSM-IV-TR, is a disorder in which individuals experience obsessions and/or compulsions. These obsessions and compulsions cause them marked distress, are time-consuming, and significantly interfere with their normal routine, occupational functioning, academic success, or social relationships. Obsessions are defined as repeated, relentless, and intrusive thoughts or images. Typical obsessions include obsessive worry about dirt or germs, periodic thoughts about something not being done properly, and discomfort that certain things must always be in a particular place. Compulsions, on the other hand, are repetitive behaviors or mental acts that affected persons feel driven to perform. Compulsions are aimed at reducing distress or at preventing some event or situation. At some point in the course of this disorder, such individuals have recognized that their obsessions or compulsions are extreme or unreasonable. Childhood-onset obsessive-compulsive disorder tends to be more common in girls, frequently runs in families, and is often accompanied by other psychiatric disorders, particularly ADHD.

40. Are problems with mood also common in children with ADHD?

Mood disorders, such as depression and bipolar disorder, are reported in anywhere from 15% to 75% of children and adolescents with ADHD.

Bipolar disorder

A mood disorder characterized by alternating depressive and manic symptoms.

Mood disorders, such as depression and **bipolar disorder**, are reported in anywhere from 15% to 75% of children and adolescents with ADHD. In a child who is depressed, the episodes of sadness go beyond the ordinary range. In other words, it is natural to be sad for short periods of time, particularly after personal losses or traumatic events. But when the sadness exceeds these normal expectations, the possibility of depression exists. Some children who are clinically depressed have physical signs, such as change in appetite or sleep patterns. Other possible symptoms include markedly diminished interest in almost all activities, fatigue or loss of energy, feelings of worthlessness, and recurrent thoughts of death. In addition, depressed children can have difficulty concentrating, just like children with ADHD. Surprisingly, some depressed children display psychomotor agitation or hyperactivity. When lack of focus or hyperactivity are involved, the distinction from ADHD can be difficult. Nevertheless, a trained professional should be able to do it. It is important to note, however, that ADHD and depression can occur simultaneously.

Bipolar disorder is another type of mood disorder. In bipolar disorder, children alternate between depressive symptoms and manic symptoms. In contrast to the depressive symptoms just described, manic symptoms may include inflated self-esteem, grandiosity, decreased need for sleep, pressured speech, racing thoughts, and excessive involvement in pleasurable activities. As with some individuals with ADHD, bipolar children may also display psychomotor agitation and be easily distracted. Similar to depression, it may at times be difficult to distinguish bipolar disorder from ADHD. In fact, many children with bipolar disorder have symptoms that would meet criteria for an ADHD diagnosis. However, some important features distinguish the two disorders. Although aggression and destructiveness are seen in both disorders, children with ADHD are often careless, whereas children with bipolar disorder may be purposefully hurtful, particularly during severe temper tantrums that may occur during more manic periods. In addition, the duration and the intensity of the outbursts differ. Outbursts are often short-lived in children with ADHD, but children with bipolar disorder can have emotional explosions that last for hours. In other words, the misbehavior in children with ADHD is often accidental, whereas bipolar children's misbehavior is often intentional.

ADHD children often are unaware of the harmful consequences of their behaviors, whereas bipolar children may be real risk seekers. In addition, both disorders may include sleep disturbances, but gruesome nightmares are sometimes seen in children with bipolar disorder. Children with bipolar disorder are also frequently gifted in particular areas and have exceptional verbal and/or artistic skills. Children with ADHD do not exhibit psychotic symptoms or loss of touch with reality. At least 85% of bipolar children show signs of false understanding of their importance, which is very uncommon in ADHD children. Rapid changes in mood are also fairly common in bipolar children.

41. Is my ADHD child's stubbornness and defiance caused by ADHD or by another condition?

Some degree of stubbornness and defiance can be normal. It is well-known that adolescents are particularly prone to these behaviors, whether or not they have ADHD. Like any other child, an ADHD child can at times be stubborn or defiant. In some instances, this falls within the normal range of behavior. However, nearly half of all children with ADHD have a comorbid oppositional defiant disorder. This disorder is characterized by negative, hostile, and defiant behavior that causes significant damage in social, academic, or occupational interactions. Children with this problem routinely argue with adults, lose their temper, and defy rules. They can be quite emotionally touchy and may blame others for their own mistakes or failures. These problems persist over time and can be quite disruptive to school, family, and social relationships.

A small percentage of children with ADHD can have a comorbid conduct disorder. In contrast to those with oppositional defiant disorder, children with conduct disorder actively transgress societal rules. Although oppositional defiant disorder is a risk factor for the later development of conduct disorder, only a small group of children with oppositional behavior eventually develop a conduct disorder. These children have serious problems at school or in the community. They take risks and break laws. In other words, they may steal, set fires, destroy property, or drive recklessly. A conduct disorder cannot be treated with medication alone. It requires intensive and ongoing therapy.

42. My ADHD child has so much trouble making and keeping friends. Is this a common problem for ADHD children?

ADHD children can be quite spontaneous and entertaining. Because of it, they may often be known as the "life of the party" or the "center of attention." However, although they may be good at stimulating interaction and attracting the attention of others, they may have more difficulty actually maintaining relationships and building appropriate friendships.

Social impairment has long been recognized as a common problem for ADHD children. In fact, many of the social difficulties experienced by ADHD children appear to be directly related to their ADHD symptoms. Thus, it could be expected that these youngsters might intrude on their peers' personal space, impulsively enter conversations, misread social cues, and be poor listeners. As executive functioning deficits are also often seen in ADHD children, cognitive rigidity, excessive talking, and dubious risk-taking behavior may occur and evoke rejection by classmates. Poor insight regarding the reasons for the ADHD's child's social difficulties may also add to the problem. Although the situation may improve with the initiation of medication, social skills training and therapeutic intervention, a very negative prior reputation and the inflexibility of peer groups may make it difficult for an ADHD child to start fresh.

Social impairment has long been recognized as a common problem for ADHD children.

43. My child had been diagnosed with an autistic spectrum disorder. My doctor now says he also has symptoms of ADHD. Can he have both?

Many children with an autistic spectrum disorder also exhibit inattention and hyperactivity that may initially be thought of as coming from internal distractions. Over time, it may become apparent that they are distracted by the external environment as well. At that point, an ADHD diagnosis should be considered and treatment options discussed.

Furthermore, some children with ADHD may also have difficulty in social situations, which is one of the three main characteristics of autistic spectrum disorder (i.e., communication problems, repetitive behaviors and restricted routines, and difficulties with social interactions). However, some children with ADHD actually have the kinds of extreme social issues that fall within the diagnostic domain of autistic spectrum disorders. These involve problems with social reciprocity and empathy, and they often manifest with poor eye contact, inflexibility and extreme reticence. One recent study assessed ADHD children with a questionnaire specifically used to diagnose autistic spectrum disorders. Autistic spectrum disorder symptoms were surprisingly common, particularly in boys with ADHD, combined type. ADHD with co-occurring autistic spectrum disorder may affect medication choices.

44. Can a child with limited intellectual capabilities have ADHD symptoms?

The major difficulty in deciding when someone with limited intellectual capabilities has ADHD trades on deciding whether to base the diagnosis on their chronological or their mental age. The criteria for ADHD per se are similar in the intellectually disabled and in children with typical development. As one would expect, the rate of diagnosis is higher when chronological age is used as the standard. Our expectations for attention, activity level, and impulse control naturally change as a child matures. Therefore, an intellectually limited 13-year-old boy may be expected to exhibit more impulsivity, poor concentration, and disorganization than intellectually normal children of the same age. However, if his distractibility, forgetfulness, fidgetiness, or inattention is excessive for what might be expected for his mental age, an ADHD diagnosis may be appropriate.

Although stimulants have been used successfully in this population, these children seem to be particularly sensitive to medications, demonstrating more side effects and sometimes requiring lower doses of their medicines. Thus, the importance of combining behavioral interventions with medications is particularly important in this population.

PART THREE

Medication and ADHD

What kinds of medication are used to treat ADHD?

Can preschoolers take stimulants? Do stimulants affect them differently?

How do I know the right time to start giving my child ADHD medication? And how long will my child need to stay on stimulants?

More . . .

45. What kinds of medication are used to treat ADHD?

The most frequently used medications for ADHD are **stimulants**, such as the methylphenidates (well-known brands are Ritalin, Focalin, Metadate, Methylin, Concerta, and Daytrana) and the amphetamines (Dexedrine, Adderall, and Vyvanse), but a number of other types of medication can be used as well. The other medications, which were often first developed to treat other medical disorders, fall into three main groups: (1) anti-tic medications, clonidine (Catapres), guanfacine (Tenex), and a new long-acting medication, Intuniv; (2) **antidepressants**; and (3) atomoxetine (Strattera), the first nonstimulant medication specifically developed for treating ADHD.

Overall, about 50% of children treated with medication for ADHD receive some form of methylphenidate (Ritalin or another brand), 30% receive some form of amphetamine (Dexedrine or Adderall), and 20% receive another type of medication.

Overall, about 50% of children treated with medication for ADHD receive some form of methylphenidate (Ritalin or another brand), 30% receive some form of amphetamine (Dexedrine or Adderall), and 20% receive another type of medication. Some receive more than one of these medications simultaneously. The pros and cons of each of the commonly used medications are discussed throughout this chapter.

THE STIMULANTS

46. I know stimulants are the most commonly prescribed medications for ADHD. Are they safe?

Stimulants are the first-choice treatment of ADHD. Stimulants have been used to treat ADHD since the 1930s. Because the stimulants have been around for many years, some adults now in their 50s and 60s remember taking medication as children. Although the information is anecdotal, there is no evidence that taking stimulant medication in childhood has caused them any long-term medical or psychological problems. More than 1000 studies have demonstrated that stimulants are safe and effective for treating the vast majority of children with properly diagnosed ADHD. Several recent studies have shown the continuing effectiveness of medication, with no apparent significant side effects even when used continually for almost a decade.

The National Institutes of Health has sponsored a large long-term Multimodal Treatment Study of Children with ADHD (the **MTA study** for short). The MTA data at year 8 was recently published; the results of the study support both the safety and probable long-term efficacy of medication. During the initial 14-month study period children receiving intensive behavioral management did not do as well with respect to the core symptoms of ADHD (inattention, hyperactivity, impulsivity) as those receiving stimulant treatment, demonstrating that medication is crucial to managing ADHD. Those children who had comorbid issues like anxiety or oppositional behavior needed both medication and behavioral management to do well. At the year 3 outcome assessment about 2 years after the study treatment protocol ended, the different treatment groups no longer differed in terms of ADHD symptoms. Those who had received intensive medication management and combined medication and behavioral management did not look better than those who had received intensive behavioral therapy or community management (whatever their private doctor prescribed). However, three subgroups (that did not correspond to the initial treatment groups) were identified at year 3: Group 1—gradual improvement over time with increasing and significant benefit from medication use at 3 years out (34% of the sample);

MTA study

National Institutes of Health-sponsored Multimodal Treatment Study of Children with ADHD.

Group 2— a larger initial improvement that was maintained over time (52% of the sample); and Group 3— returned to baseline symptoms after initial benefit (14% of the sample). Thus, while all the expected benefits were not present at year 3, most of the children were doing well. Intensive medication management may only make a persistent long-term difference if it is continued with the same intensity as during the MTA's initial 14-month study period. In contrast, starting or adding medication at a less than optimal intensity and/or too late in a child's ADHD clinical course (particularly if a child's behavior is deteriorating) may not only be ineffective but also (if not carefully examined in data analysis) even make medication appear to be associated with worse outcomes. Some children may eventually be able to stop medication perhaps just because they were intensively treated early on. Medication alone and combined therapy did decrease the number of ADHD children who developed oppositional defiant disorder at the 3-year follow-up.

Other data show that stimulant medications do not have any adverse effects on brain development. There are minor differences in the size of certain brain areas in ADHD children compared to children without ADHD, but these are present prior to medication use. After medication is begun, these structures continue to enlarge on the same trajectory as in non-ADHD children. But, they remain approximately 5% smaller than in the non-ADHD child.

Perhaps more than any other medicines, stimulants seem to suffer from "bad press"—most likely related to the public's unfounded blurring of the distinctions between stimulants as medication and as drugs of abuse. Given the large number of children and the families potentially affected, efforts to help the public to understand these distinctions are extremely important. Stimulants, used as prescribed, are not addictive. Furthermore, children treated with stimulants are less likely to be substance abusers later in life than are ADHD children who have not been treated with stimulants.

47. Are the stimulants overprescribed?

Another concern, again unfounded, is that stimulants are overprescribed. In the mid-1990s, the number of prescriptions in the United States for Ritalin and other stimulants for ADHD children was 2.5 times as high as in 1990. (We often use Ritalin in this book to stand in for all stimulant medication.) The number of prescriptions has continued to climb. This increase has aroused concern that stimulants are being overprescribed. However, the increased number of prescriptions is consistent with a current conservative estimate of the frequency of ADHD in children as 4% to 5%. The increase in prescriptions, therefore, is due to several factors, including the heightened awareness of the disorder, the increase in the diagnosis of ADHD in girls, increased recognition of the inattentive subtype of ADHD, and the continuation or start of treatment in adolescence and adulthood. Also, the use of stimulant medication has increased in preschoolers during this same period. More Ritalin is being prescribed in other countries as well (e.g., Britain).

Yet, in spite of these increases, not all children with ADHD are properly diagnosed, and not all children with ADHD are properly treated. In other words, in some instances Ritalin is actually being underprescribed. Data from four different communities indicates that only one of every eight 9- to 17-year-olds diagnosed with ADHD had ever received stimulant medication treatment.

48. How do stimulants affect the brain? How can they help an already overstimulated child? Isn't that paradoxical?

Stimulant medications increase brain levels of dopamine, and to a lesser extent norepinephrine and serotonin, particularly in the frontal and striatal regions.

Stimulant medications increase brain levels of dopamine, and to a lesser extent norepinephrine and serotonin, particularly in the frontal and striatal regions. A person who does not have ADHD and has a normally functioning frontal cortex experiences a medication induced increase in dopamine as a very modest increase in focus. Persons who have ADHD and an underfunctioning frontal cortex experience increased dopamine—which results from stimulants—in very much the same way, but the effects are much more dramatic. Improved frontal functioning means that other parts of their brain can stop overcompensating. Freed from excess activity in the rest of the brain and with a sudden ability to focus, children with ADHD feel calmer than before and so may be less hyperactive. Furthermore, they are more attentive, less easily distracted, and less impulsive.

In one study of non-ADHD adults, Ritalin increased their interest in performing a mathematics task. Increased interest may be one of the reasons why the drug improves school performance in children with ADHD. The increase in the interest for the mathematics tasks seen with Ritalin was associated with an increase in dopamine in the brain, especially in the striatum, as measured by functional imaging.

Stimulants work throughout the frontal striatal circuit. Ritalin and Dexedrine, although they are slightly different chemically, have similar effects. They increase dopamine levels in the synaptic area. Ritalin blocks the dopamine transporter, an enzyme that scoops up dopamine from the synaptic region and transports it back into the presynaptic neuron, and to a lesser degree promotes release of dopamine from storage vesicles in the presynaptic neuron. Dexedrine's primary action is to release dopamine from storage vesicles in the presynaptic neuron. It reverses the dopamine transporter function to a lesser degree than does Ritalin, but increases the amount of dopamine in the synaptic space to a similar degree (see Questions 7 and 8).

Although ADHD is probably primarily a disorder of dopamine metabolism, norepinephrine and even serotonin play a role. The balance between dopamine and these latter two neurotransmitters may also be an aspect of the disorder. Both Ritalin and Dexedrine affect norepinephrine and serotonin levels as well, but to a lesser degree than they affect dopamine. The involvement of norepinephrine and serotonin in ADHD probably explains why other medications are useful for treating this disorder.

49. How effective are stimulant medications, and how do I know whether they are working?

A positive response to stimulants occurs in 70% to 80% of children with ADHD treated with these medications. (A response to stimulant medications is not, however, proof that the diagnosis is ADHD.) The use of stimulant medications results in an immediate and often dramatic improvement in behavior. Attentiveness improves and interpersonal interactions are enhanced. Teachers do not need to work as hard to control a child in the classroom and are more approving of their behavior. Scores on laboratory measures of attention, impulsivity, learning, information processing, short-term memory,

A positive response to stimulants occurs in 70% to 80% of children with ADHD treated with these medications.

and vigilance are all enhanced. Academic performance in both the short- and long-term improves as well.

Stimulant medications are reported to be effective in patients of all ages, from preschool children to adults. Characteristics such as race, gender, family income, and parents' marital status do not predict treatment response. Generally, it is clear when stimulants are working. Your child should be less fidgety, more focused, better able to stay on task, and less impulsive. Optimally, people who do not know your child is taking medication should comment on the change. You, your child, and your child's teachers should all notice when medication is missed. Also, your child should detect and appreciate the differences produced by medication.

Studies show that parents and teachers generally agree on whether a child is responding to medication. However, monitoring school ratings is important, because ADHD symptoms often come to light in more cognitively challenging settings or in settings where individuals have less control over task selection (i.e., at school). Questionnaires completed by parents, teachers, and youths before and after treatment are the most commonly used method to check the effectiveness of medication. Sometimes, repeating certain parts of neuropsychological testing is helpful to determine the effectiveness of medication and to fine-tune the dosage.

50. What different kinds of stimulants are available? What are their advantages and disadvantages?

The biggest differences between stimulants have to do with how long they last. This, in turn, has to do with how they are packaged. Stimulant differences may also reflect slight differences in effects on the neurotransmitters involved in ADHD.

All doctors have their own style of managing ADHD medications; there is no "cookbook" formula. Many start with short-acting forms of medicine and then move to long-acting forms on the basis of a child's response. In one typical scenario, the starting dose of standard Ritalin or Adderall is 5 mg once daily. Your doctors may increase the dose every few days while they monitor your child's behavior and academic performance using reports from you, the teachers, and even your child. Your doctor should be asking about side effects as well. When doctors arrive at the optimal dose, they can determine the length of time for which the medicine is effective and can assess the need for, the timing of, and the type of additional doses. Definite individual differences are found in "kick-in time," time of maximum effect, and duration of effect. In other words, the same stimulant at the same dose can affect two children very differently.

The same stimulant at the same dose can affect two children very differently.

Some doctors start immediately with a long-acting preparation, particularly in older children with long school days and lots of homework. "Ballpark" doses of medications range from 1 to 2 mg/kg of body weight/day for Ritalin to 0.5 to 1 mg/kg of body weight/day for Dexedrine–Adderall–Focalin. Some children **metabolize** the medicines quickly and need higher doses; others metabolize them slowly and need lower doses. The dose does not necessarily reflect the severity of the problem. If a child is on a "high" dose but metabolizes it quickly, he probably ends up with the same amount of medicine in his system as the child who metabolizes a "regular" dose at the standard rate. Older, bigger children do not

Metabolize

What the body does in reaction to a medication. Some people are relatively fast and some people are relatively slow metabolizers. This means that people can require different doses of the same medication to get similar effects.

necessarily need higher doses because metabolism may slow down as they hit the teen years.

Because some children will respond to Ritalin family medicines and not to Adderall family medicines and vice versa, trying the other brand is usually worthwhile if the first one does not work. About half the time, children respond equally well to Ritalin or Adderall. However, about one-fourth respond better to one than to the other. Even different name brands of the same stimulant may affect the same child differently. Thus, trying more than one is well worth the effort.

Beth's comment:

Jane took a stimulant for several months and had a really positive response at school. However, she complained that she felt less spontaneous when taking the medication. At an office visit, the doctor suggested that she try a different brand-name stimulant. Jane noticed an immediate, positive difference. Her father, who knew nothing about the medication change, commented during that first week that Jane was bubbling and talkative, but nonetheless quite focused.

Although school personnel and teachers need to be told that your child is taking medication, sometimes starting medication without telling them can be helpful in determining your child's response while avoiding a bias about medication that may go in either direction. This may be impossible if the child needs a dose during the school day, which would be administered by the school nurse, but if not, it can provide an opportunity to "test" the effects. In the best of all possible worlds, the teachers of a student starting on stimulants will report an outstanding week. Another way to decide the effectiveness of stimulants in the absence of any bias is to determine—on occasions when a dose of the stimulant has been missed or skipped—whether your child's behavior and school performance decline dramatically.

The time of year in which your child receives an ADHD diagnosis can affect a medication start-up plan. Doctors and parents may hurry to medicate children who are first given a diagnosis in the spring to get them ready for finals, or try to use a shorter trial period to plan for the following school year. You can try out medication over vacations and in the summer, but ensuring what response your child will have at school is harder. You will then find out whether there are any negative effects.

Never try out a new medication on an important school day. Adjusting medications for special situations requires planning. For example, your child may benefit from a medicine regimen for taking important morning examinations (e.g., finals or SATs) that differs from that for a regular school day. Simulating "the real thing" on different trial doses can be helpful. Long final examinations occurring in the afternoon may also require preplanned medication adjustments.

Each of the different kinds of stimulant preparations has advantages and disadvantages. Short-acting stimulant preparations provide for more flexibility. Some children need a short-acting form of the medicine on their night table to take as soon as they wake up. They need it for the morning home routines. Some high school and college students prefer short-acting medications that they can adjust, depending on their varying daily schedule. They can use short-acting preparations in addition to long-acting medications to maximize the effect at a particular time (e.g., early in the morning or for homework and independent study). Short-acting preparations are

Short-acting stimulant preparations provide for more flexibility.

Rebound

Irritability, moodiness, fatigue, or hyperactivity as medicine wears off.

more often associated with **rebound** (irritability, moodiness, fatigue, or hyperactivity as the medicine wears off) than are long-acting preparations. However, that does not mean that rebound will necessarily occur.

Intermediate-acting stimulants provide a different kind of flexibility. They might be particularly useful in the elementary school-age children who need coverage only through early afternoon and who do not get much homework. Kick-in time is relatively rapid. Rebound should be less than with the short-acting drugs.

ADHD children generally can take the long-acting drugs once a day. Even a 10-day course of antibiotics can be a chore, so imagine how hard it is to take medication every single day—even just once a day. Although the long-acting medicines may cover the school day, they may not last long enough to cover homework time, particularly for older students who do homework or study in the late evening. Higher doses of the long-acting stimulants tend to last longer. Some children may need a long-acting form of medicine initially and a short- or intermediate-acting, or even another long-acting form of medicine in the late afternoon to cover the late afternoon and evening homework period. During less-structured homework time, some children may actually need medication even more than they do during school. Even if parents are going to sit and work with their children on a one-to-one basis, medication may facilitate the process. For some children, both short- and long-acting medications may have to be given together in the morning to help them to be less impulsive on the school bus and more focused for first period at school.

Long-acting stimulant medicines also have non-school–related advantages. Adolescents drive more carefully when they have taken medication (discussed in Question 97). The effects of the stimulants during the late afternoon and early evening may decrease impulsivity and help teenagers to stay out of trouble. Another obvious advantage of long-acting drugs is that affected children need not go to the school nurse to receive medications. They retain their privacy, which is especially important during the sometimes difficult adolescent years.

The long-acting medications also generally eliminate the rebound effect seen in some children when short-acting preparations wear off abruptly. Long-acting medications kick in more slowly and also dissipate more smoothly. The long-acting preparations vary in the timing of their maximum and minimum effects (**Tables 3** and **4**). For example, most children with ADHD may behave better at school than at home if they take Ritalin LA in the morning instead of Concerta. Ritalin LA takes effect faster but does not last as long. Sometimes children on Concerta need to take a short-acting preparation together with the Concerta to cover their bus ride and first class. However, if children take Concerta, improvements in behavior generally last longer, covering the period after school and the early evening homework time. Children on Ritalin LA or Adderall XR may need to take a booster of short- or intermediate-acting medicine to cover homework time. Vyvanse, a new formulation of Adderall, generally lasts through the day into the evening. Vyvanse is a prodrug and is not activated until it is in the stomach. (Thus, it cannot be abused.) The Daytrana patch (which contains Ritalin) works for up to 12 hours (**Figure 4**). The child removes the patch 3 hours before he/she wants the stimulant effect to stop. The patch can be used for short days too. For example, you can remove it after 4 hours and get the effect of medication for a total of 7 hours.

The long-acting medications also generally eliminate the rebound effect seen in some children when short-acting preparations wear off abruptly.

Table 3   Medications Commonly Used to Treat ADHD

Drug	Starts to Work	Peak Effect	Average Duration of Effect	Number of Dose per Day	Usual Dose Range (mg)
Ritalin, Methylin	30–60 min	2 hr	3–5 hr	2–3	5–60 mg of Ritalin, but 80 mg has been used by practitioners
Dexedrine, Dextrostat	30–60 min	1–3 hr	3–6 hr	2–3	5–40
Adderall	30–60 min	1–2 hr	4–6 hr	2	5–30, sometimes 40
Focalin	30–60 min	60–90 min	4–6 hr	2	5–20, Focalin dose 1/2 of the Ritalin dose
Ritalin SR, Methylin ER	60–90 min	5 hr (1.5–6)	5–8 hr	2	5–60
Dexedrine spantule	60–90 min	3–4 hr	5–8 hr	2	10–40
Ritalin LA, Metadate OD	30 min to 2 hr	2 peaks (1–3 hr, 6 hr, 1.5 hr, 4.5 hr)	6–10 hr	1–2	10–60
Concerta	30 min to 2 hr	3 peaks (2 hr, 6–8 hr)	10–12 hr; increasing dose may increase duration of effect	1	18–54, but 100 mg has been used by practitioners
Adderall XR	1–2 hr	3 peaks (2 hr, 6–8 hr)	10–12 hr; increasing dose may increase duration of effect	1	5–60
Focalin XR	30 min to 2 hr	2 peaks (2 hr, 8 hr)	10–12 hr	1	5–20, usually 1/2 of the Ritalin dose
Daytrana patch	1–2 hr	Steady effect	12 hr, patch worn for 9 hrs, benefit continues for 3 hours after patch removed	1	10–30, dose usually about 1/2 of Ritalin dose
Vyvance	1 hr	Steady effect	12	1	30–70

Note: Methylphenidate is the generic name for Ritalin, Focalin, Metadate, Methylin, and Concerta. Amphetamine is the generic name for Dexedrine and Adderall.

Table 4   Effect of Medications on Different Neurotransmitters

	Serotonin	Norepinephrine	Dopamine
Stimulants			
Ritalin			Increases ++++
Dexedrine-Adderall	Increases +	Increases ++	Increases ++++
Strattera		Increases +++	Increases +
Nonstimulants			
Tricyclic antidepressants	Increases ++	Increases + to +++, depending on brand	
Wellbutrin		Increases ++	Increases ++
Effexor	Low dose increases ++	Midsize dose increases ++	High dose increases ++
Catapres, Tenex		Increases ++	
Selective serotonin reuptake inhibitors (SSRIs)	Increases +++		

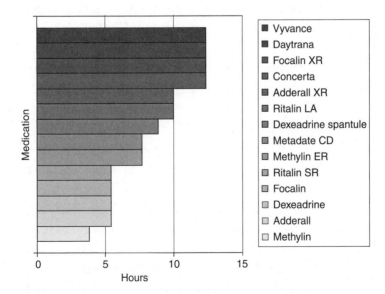

Figure 4   Duration of Action of Various ADHD Medications.

51. What effects do stimulants and other ADHD medications have on brain neurotransmitters? What behaviors do neurotransmitters affect?

The different medications currently used to treat ADHD affect the three major neurotransmitters (dopamine, norepinephrine, and serotonin) to differing degrees, that is, increasing the levels of the neurotransmitters in the brain. This in turn affects behavior. But there is not always a reason explaining the behavioral response in comparison with the biochemical response.

Dopamine is the neurotrans- mitter most relevant to ADHD.

Dopamine is the neurotransmitter most relevant to ADHD. Dopamine functions in many different ways in the brain. It plays a key role in motor control. For example, dopamine levels are low in Parkinson's disease, where difficulties controlling movement are the primary symptom. Atypical dopamine function may play a role in the hyperactivity seen in ADHD individuals. Dopamine also plays a role in reward-oriented behaviors; thus, abnormal dopamine function may also play a role in the impulsivity seen in ADHD.

Dopamine levels affect pleasurable feelings, so much so that it has been called the "pleasure neurotransmitter." Many natural activities trigger an increase in brain dopamine. Dopamine is released during everyday enjoyable activities such as reading a good book, listening to music, or participating in sports. In those instances dopamine neurons release dopamine and produce a natural good feeling. Drugs can also trigger dopamine release. Cocaine very rapidly increases dopamine levels in the brain, which is why it produces a "high." Stimulant medications also increase dopamine levels, but over hours rather than immediately. This difference in the rate of dopamine release is the difference between the increase in dopamine causing extremely pleasurable highs (cocaine) and dopamine acting to increase focus and attention (stimulants). However, what should be noted is that stimulants taken in ways not prescribed, such as snorted or taken intravenously, also increase dopamine levels rapidly and produce a high. Such misuse can be harmful, which is why some parents worry about giving ADHD drugs to children (see Question 57). Thus, it is important to be aware of the need to follow the prescribing doctor and/or pharmacist's instructions carefully and to monitor your child's use of the prescription.

52. What are the side effects of stimulant medications?

By and large, the side effects of stimulants, if they occur at all, are nuisance side effects. Studies looking at side effects suggest minimal differences between stimulant medications and **placebo** (fake pills with no medication in them). This means that most of the time, side effects are coincidental and are not actually related to the medication itself. Some side effects that have been described include headache, dizziness, trouble sleeping, stomach aches, and poor appetite. These side effects do not happen to everybody; indeed, they do not happen to most children. Many times, even if they do occur, they are short-lived.

Placebo

"Sugar pills" used in a clinical trial to identify whether the subject is responding just to the act of taking a pill or to the medication being tested.

Effects on the Heart

Mild increases in heart rate and blood pressure are sometimes seen, but are not a health risk. Nevertheless, your child's heart rate and blood pressure should be routinely checked. There is no evidence that an EKG or cardiac workup is needed before trying stimulants. If, however, there is a family history of sudden unexplained death in a young adult, your doctor will probably send your child to a cardiologist to be evaluated for a rare cardiac disorder—idiopathic hypertrophic cardiomyopathy. An echocardiogram (a picture of the heart) is required to rule this out.

Appetite Suppression

Approximately 80% of ADHD children taking stimulant medication report decreased appetite, but often it is mild and limited to lunchtime eating. Catch-up eating occurs after school and in the evening, so children get the calories and nutrition they need. Rarely, after-school medications interfere at dinner time, but shifting meal time around a little can take care of this. Unless your child is losing weight or gaining weight poorly, you should not consider a minor decrease in appetite an issue. Finding breakfast foods and lunch foods your child likes to eat should be your priority. Here, enjoyment may take precedence over nutritional status. Some children experience more appetite suppression from one stimulant than from another, so trying several is worth the effort if appetite suppression is bothersome. Obviously, monitoring weight regularly is important. Vitamin supplements are never a bad idea either.

Personality Changes

Personality change from stimulant medication can be an issue on rare occasions. Some children do become less spontaneous on medication. The degree to which that happens, how such children and their parents feel about it, and how effective the medication is all factor into the decision about what to do. Sometimes switching to a different stimulant helps; sometimes a medication from a different family of drugs is needed. Producing a "zombie"-like child to satisfy a teacher is obviously not acceptable. However, most children remain "themselves" in personality (minus the behavioral problems) while on medication. Occasionally, children report effects of medication on their personality only in specific circumstances. Some children find medicine inhibiting when they play sports; others find it enhances their performance because they focus better. Timing medicine properly can take care of many of these issues.

Insomnia

Insomnia has been reported in anywhere from 3% to 85% of children with ADHD. Although an occasional child has trouble with sleep as a side effect of stimulant medications, many ADHD children have trouble with sleeping as a chronic long-term problem that arose before any medication use. Many such children describe an inability to settle down and to stop thinking at bedtime. Other events of daily life that can interfere with falling asleep are uncompleted homework, exciting television shows, video games, bedtime fears, or loneliness in addition to oppositional tendencies. Behavioral management is helpful here. In some children, stimulants may actually decrease sleep problems by minimizing distracting thoughts. For many children, moderate afternoon exercise, maintaining consistent bedtime routines, and relaxation strategies in bed will help them to sleep.

Some studies have suggested that children with ADHD are more likely to have allergies than children who do not have ADHD. Some children with allergies have difficulty falling asleep because their allergies act up at nighttime. Sometimes, giving allergy medications—which can be sedating—at bedtime may provide a two-for-one benefit.

Sleep delays of about an hour or more can be debilitating and result in excessive daytime sleepiness. This can worsen a child's problems with attention. So, on occasion, medication may be necessary to improve sleep.

For example, clonidine (discussed in Question 66), a medication used to treat ADHD—particularly the element of hyperactivity—may also be useful at bedtime to improve sleep. It can be used in combination with stimulants. Melatonin, (which has now been manufactured by pharmaceutical companies), the hormone that the brain produces naturally at nighttime as a signal that it is time to sleep, can also be used about an hour before bedtime to promote sleep.

Staying asleep is another common problem for ADHD children whether they are taking stimulants or not. Nighttime enuresis (bedwetting) can awaken children. Nighttime enuresis tends to last longer in ADHD children than in children without ADHD. This problem can be managed by eliminating fluids after dinner. Sometimes medications are necessary in situations in which bedwetting is embarrassing (e.g., at camp or during sleepovers). DDAVP (which has also now been manufactured by pharmaceutical companies) is the hormone that the brain produces to prevent urination. It is administered as a nasal spray before bedtime. Restless leg syndrome occurs with increased frequency in children with ADHD. It is a sleep disorder characterized by leg discomfort during sleep, which is only relieved by frequent movements of the legs. Thus, sleep can be interrupted with resulting day time sleepiness accentuating already compromised attention. Some children with restless leg syndrome are iron deficient, and iron supplements may help treat restless leg syndrome.

Note that depression can cause difficulties with falling asleep and can cause early morning awakening. Because depression can occur as a comorbid disorder with ADHD or can simulate ADHD, one should give this possibility careful consideration.

Growth

Parents should monitor growth in children taking stimulants. Whether stimulant medications affect growth in children has been a subject of debate. Overall, the studies to date document that the long-term effects are minimal and are not of clinical importance. It is fair to say that stimulant-treated children end up as tall as their parents. However, you should routinely measure your child's height.

Most physicians do not do routine blood testing in children taking stimulants, but some do. Your pediatrician probably checks blood count and perhaps blood chemistries at your child's yearly checkup. This is sufficient.

53. Can children with tics take stimulant medications? Can stimulants cause tics or Tourette's?

ADHD and tics and Tourette's (defined as motor and vocal tics that last longer than 1 year with no periods of remission) are all fairly common childhood problems. They often run in the same family and can be caused by the same gene(s). Tics and Tourette's can occur in as many as 25% of children with ADHD, and ADHD occurs in the majority of children with Tourette's (see Question 37). Because of older reports that suggested a causal relationship between stimulants and tics–Tourette's, questions have been raised about the best way to use stimulants in children with tics–Tourette's and what to do if tics appear while an ADHD child is taking stimulants. None of the placebo-controlled, **double-blind, cross-over studies** have shown a significant increase in tics resulting from stimulant treatment in children with ADHD and tics–Tourette's, nor

Double-blind

A study in which neither the subject nor the investigator know whether the subject is getting the drug or the placebo.

Cross-over study

A study in which the subject takes one treatment for part of the study period and another treatment for the other part of the study period. Usually one treatment is the drug being tested and the other treatment is a placebo.

have the prospective follow-up studies of children who had tics–Tourette's at the outset or whose tics appeared during stimulant treatment. Increases in tics or the appearance of tics in children who have never had tics are relatively common during the placebo phase of controlled studies. This suggests that in at-risk children, changes in their environment—even just taking a new pill—can provoke a reaction. Because ADHD tends to present 2 to 3 years before tics–Tourette's, the appearance of tics–Tourette's may mistakenly be attributed to the stimulant medications used to treat ADHD rather than to the presence of comorbid ADHD and Tourette's. When tics do occur in children taking stimulant medications, they have tended to be relatively mild and often transient, and have rarely required that stimulants be stopped.

Despite the careful clinical studies, our increased knowledge of the genetic relationship between ADHD and tics–Tourette's, and a clearer picture of the natural history of tics–Tourette's, the management of tics–Tourette's in ADHD children taking stimulants is not always clear-cut. Rarely do children have a significant increase of tics when taking stimulant medication. Sometimes, the worsened condition is related to the dose of stimulants, and lowering the dose takes care of the problem. Sometimes, significant tic increases occur after use of one stimulant but not another. Additionally, in some children with tics–Tourette's and ADHD, the tics definitely diminish when they are treated with stimulants! Rarely is the tic increase bad enough to require the addition of an anti-tic medication or to discontinue stimulants. Notably, in a recent study of children with Tourette's and ADHD, the best outcome in all respects, including the area of academics, was in a group receiving both stimulants and an anti-tic medication (clonidine, discussed in Question 66). Individualized therapy or biofeedback (or both) may also be useful in treating symptoms in children with ADHD and tics–Tourette's.

54. Can preschoolers take stimulants? Do stimulants affect them differently?

Yes, doctors can use stimulants to treat preschoolers with ADHD. Clearly, in young children the pros and cons of medication must be weighed with particular care. On the one hand, children receiving an ADHD diagnosis as preschoolers may have more severe problems and therefore should be medicated more liberally. Because the range of acceptable behaviors is obviously broader for preschool children, those who stand out in the crowd generally have very significant problems. On the other hand, that broad range makes correct diagnosis harder. One must never take medication use in young children lightly. A percentage of children who appear to have ADHD as preschoolers outgrow the diagnosis in elementary school. Therefore, careful follow-up of preschoolers taking medication is mandatory.

Although some studies suggest a response rate equal to that of older children, other studies find that preschool children are less responsive to stimulant treatment and have more side effects. Possibly the high rates of comorbidity of mood and anxiety disorders and conduct disorders in preschoolers create more complex situations and make treating preschoolers more difficult. Because hyperactivity is a prominent symptom in preschool children and the degree of attentiveness required is not as high as that of schoolage children, such medications as clonidine or guanfacine (discussed in Question 66) are often used to treat ADHD in preschoolers. In contrast to stimulant medications, they have their most

Studies find that preschool children are less responsive to stimulant treatment and have more side effects.

marked effect on hyperactive and impulsive behavior and a lesser effect on attention per se.

55. Do stimulant medications improve social skills?

Yes, improved social interactions can be an important benefit. Children with ADHD often stand out in the crowd. Not only their teachers but their peers notice them. Their peers are less likely to want to sit next to them or to name them as a best friend. Studies show that ADHD children who are taking medications are more popular and better liked than those who are not medicated. High ratings by peers in social areas are excellent predictors of success in later life. So, improving the social abilities of children with ADHD—which medication does—is an investment in their future.

Although it makes intuitive sense to assume that social skills and better cooperation with parents require explicit teaching, the National Institutes of Health sponsored Multimodal Treatment Study of Children with ADHD study findings (Question 46) suggests that many children can often acquire these abilities when medication takes care of their ADHD symptoms. This suggests that core symptoms of ADHD (e.g., being impulsive and hyperactive) may interfere with learning specific social skills. Thus, medication may benefit many children in areas not previously considered to be medication targets.

You should not crush, or let your child chew, the sustained- or extended-release formulations.

56. How do I give stimulant medications to my child?

You should not crush, or let your child chew, the sustained- or extended-release formulations (Ritalin SR, Ritalin LA, Metadate CD, Methylin ER, Concerta, Adderall XR, Dexedrine spantule, Vyvanse). Your child should swallow these whole with water or some other drink. They are designed to release medication slowly in the body. However, if your child can not swallow a pill, there are certain brands that you can open (Ritalin LA, Metadate CD, and Adderall XR capsules) and sprinkle into a tablespoon of food at room temperature (e.g., applesauce). You should use the mixture immediately. Do not save it for later. If in doubt, ask your pharmacist.

Food intake affects the time it takes for medication to start to work. Food can affect some stimulants more than it affects others. Concerta is least affected by food. Other intermediate- and long-acting drugs begin to work more slowly when taken on a full stomach, especially a high-fat meal or one with citrus fruits. However, you must strike a balance between getting a good breakfast and the "kick-in time" for the medication. Generally, the best policy is to take the medication in the same way every day, before, with, or after meals.

A quick "kick" of medication in the morning is important to help a child focus on everyday tasks. Morning chores such as brushing teeth, getting dressed, or organizing a backpack can be extremely tedious and difficult for the ADHD child to complete. Medications can help if they're timed properly. Stimulants also help in unstructured situations. The bus ride to school, for example, is often a free-for-all, especially if it is long—a situation that is not uncommon, because children with ADHD may have learning disabilities that require special schooling far away. Effective medications levels can help in these situations.

If your child misses a dose, give him the missed dose as soon as you remember. However, if you do not remember until you are close to the time the next dose is due or it is already evening, skip the missed dose and administer only the next regularly scheduled dose. Do not give your child a double dose of his or her medication, unless your doctor tells you to do so.

If you think that you may have accidentally given—or your child may have intentionally or unintentionally taken—too much medication, check with your doctor right away. If your child has taken an unknown amount, seek medical attention immediately. From 1993 to 1999, about 13,000 overdoses were reported to poison control centers; 2,500 were reported in 1999. The increasing frequency of Ritalin "overdose" parallels increasing use. The majority of children experienced no effect (60%) or experienced minor effects (30%). No fatalities have occurred. The most common reasons for overdose were unintentional errors in children younger than 13 and suicide attempts in adolescents. Adolescents were more likely to experience side effects, require hospitalizations, and have more serious complications.

Symptoms of a stimulant overdose include agitation, tremors, muscle twitches, seizures, confusion, hallucinations, sweating, flushing, headache, fast or irregular heartbeat, large pupils, and dryness of the mouth and eyes. The difference between the dose for treatment and the dose causing these kinds of effects is usually rather large. Double doses, giving medication twice by mistake, are unlikely to cause overdose symptoms.

57. If my child refuses to take ADHD medication, what can I do?

Parents of ADHD children need to have serious discussions with them about the nature of their disorder and why it is important to treat it. A parent can compare

ADHD to other chronic illnesses, such as asthma or diabetes, where daily medicines are required. Try comparing the pills to eyeglasses, braces, or allergy medication, and remind the child that they are lucky that medications are available to help them do better in school, experience fewer problems with peers, and generally get along better in life. The child's doctor should talk with him or her as well. Sometimes, coming up with a trial plan in which such children feel that they have some control helps to get them to start medication. Then, if medicine works, hopefully resistance becomes a moot point. If it does not, you may consider bringing your child to a counselor who specializes in children with ADHD or learning disabilities; the resistance may stem from fears of being "different" or other emotional concerns that can be resolved with counseling.

It is important to remain low key and not turn the medication into a subject for argument. Make sure the child understands that the medication is being offered to benefit him, not the parents or the teachers. If your child senses anxiety on your part over whether he or she takes the medication, it may become a weapon in a battle of wills should conflict arise between you, even if the argument starts over an unrelated subject. This is especially true of adolescents, who are constantly trying to assume greater autonomy and are more resistant to parental control.

58. I find the idea of giving my child medication very worrisome. Can my child become dependent on or addicted to stimulants?

No parents want to give their child medication, even for such small things as colds and coughs. However, if your child has a medical problem, the only treatment that is truly effective is medication. If your child has a strep throat, you may not be thrilled, but you would use antibiotics because medically the situation calls for antibiotics. Negative media coverage of stimulants and its effect on public opinion may unfortunately prevent as many as one-half of ADHD children from being treated properly.

Proponents of medication argue that Ritalin and related medications have been extensively studied and are quite safe when properly monitored. Failure to treat ADHD properly may worsen a problematic situation by delaying developmental progress, thereby increasing the likelihood of low self-esteem, social problems, and educational difficulties. Opponents of medication suggest that the rise in stimulant use results either from physicians feeling pressured by pharmaceutical companies to write more prescriptions or from physicians and parents who do not have the time (or the will) to seek out alternative forms of treatment that do not involve medication. Some even claim that parents who do not wish to deal with a growing child's energy would rather "have the child diagnosed" so they can medicate the child's energy away rather than channel it into sports or other physical activities. Unfortunately, this idea results from the failure to understand that ADHD is a biochemical problem, and not simply a product of a child's natural energy, high spirits, or a desire to get attention. Most parents and doctors turn to medications only when the child's difficulties create a serious disruption in the child's daily life. The bottom line is that you cannot simply "train" a child, as you would an energetic puppy, to focus and pay attention if the neurotransmitters are out of balance. To change the behavior, you must address the chemical imbalance in the brain, and that requires medication.

Failure to treat ADHD properly may worsen a problematic situation by delaying developmental progress, thereby increasing the likelihood of low self-esteem, social problems, and educational difficulties.

Because medication produces such dramatic effects, most parents grow to be quite accepting of using medication. Most studies show that children and adolescents generally feel okay about taking medication. Of course, they take their cue to some degree from their families. If you view ADHD as a medical problem that, like diabetes, requires medical treatment, your child will too. One of the goals of the MTA study (see Question 46) was to compare the medication treatment with other forms of treatment. Children who received medication expertly managed by the study researchers with or without behavioral therapy did better than those who received very extensive behavioral therapy alone. When you have a biochemical problem, nothing really substitutes for medication.

Parents often feel overwhelmed when it comes to deciding whether to give medication to their child for ADHD. Thinking about the following questions may help you to figure out what's best for your child. Some of these questions can be answered without consulting a medical expert. Others will require you to consult with professionals involved with your child's care (e.g., teacher, counselor, psychologist, or physician).

- About what behaviors are you concerned?
- Are these behaviors manageable? At home? At school?
- Do these behaviors interfere with your child's functioning? At home? At school? Among friends?
- About what behaviors is the school concerned? Do they affect academics? Do they affect social interactions?
- Are you concerned about your child's safety?
- With what approaches or treatments are your child, your family, and you comfortable?
- What are the risks of medication?

- What are the risks of not using medication?
- How do your child, your family, and you feel about the idea of your child taking medication?

Many parents worry that they are teaching their children to take drugs by giving them stimulant medications. But more and more studies suggest that children who have ADHD and do not get treated are more likely to abuse illicit drugs than are children who take medication. Furthermore, when children are taking the proper medication, they are less impulsive, more attentive, and more socially careful. Your child is actually better equipped to refuse illicit drugs because he can stop and carefully consider the consequences rather than act on impulse.

Your child may depend on stimulants to help performance in school and overcome ADHD symptoms, but he will not become physically dependent on or addicted to stimulants. ADHD children can take "drug holidays" (discussed in Question 61) with no physical ill effects. True drug **dependence** produces a physical need for a drug; withdrawal symptoms appear if the drug is stopped. This is true for prescribed medications as well as for drugs of abuse that produce a high. However, you do not become physically dependent on stimulant medications when they are used properly. Some children seem to need increasingly higher doses. Some of these children may be depressed and in a sense be using the stimulant to self-medicate based on the mild antidepressant effect of stimulants.

Dependence

The physical need for the repeatedly used abused drug to the point where withdrawal symptoms will appear if the drug is stopped.

Stimulants actually are not that easily abused. Taken orally, they produce the same effect on focus in someone abusing them (albeit to a lesser degree) as they do for someone who uses them for ADHD. Taken in larger-than-normal doses by someone with or without ADHD, they can cause agitation and anxiety. Palpitations may occur, but you do not get "high." There is no apparent benefit. Taken regularly in extremely large doses, stimulants can produce hallucinations and paranoid behavior as well as dramatic mood swings. No real reason to abuse them exists—unless you are looking for enhanced focus and concentration, for example, to stay up late and finish a paper. Children with ADHD may stay up late to finish homework or papers, but they do not tend to use their stimulants late at night just to stay awake. Indeed, they sometimes do not use them when they should.

To better understand why they are not addictive, it might help to contrast the effects of stimulants with the effects of crack-cocaine, which is being increasingly abused because it produces explosive, pleasurable highs. Cocaine has this effect because it causes very rapid increases in brain levels of dopamine (discussed in Question 51). This occurs because users inhale or inject cocaine, which then is rapidly absorbed into their bloodstream and travels quickly to their brain. Stimulant medications, however, are taken orally. They are absorbed very gradually into the bloodstream and build up slowly in the brain. Although they (like cocaine) release dopamine, they do so at a much slower rate. The rate of increase of dopamine is what determines whether a drug produces a high, and it is the high that makes cocaine addictive. If you were to crush a tablet of a stimulant medication and inhale or inject it, your dopamine brain levels would rise more quickly, and you could get high. You could conceivably become psychologically dependent and even physically addicted. Of course, you can do that also by sniffing airplane glue, paint thinner, and gasoline, if you really want to get high. The point is, medications used properly and as prescribed pose no danger to your child.

Medications used properly and as prescribed pose no danger to your child.

Another point of concern for parents is the relationship between amphetamines such as Dexedrine to "speed." Methamphetamine (the real "speed") sold on the street does have chemical similarities to stimulants like Dexedrine. All amphetamines share some biochemical properties, just as opiate derivatives like codeine or morphine share qualities with heroin but clearly are not the same drug. However, the abuse potential of speed versus stimulants is very different. Even the abuse potential of oral methamphetamine is relatively low. In a study looking at the effects of methamphetamine speed in normal volunteers, only two rated their response as positive ("I feel a good drug effect" and "I feel high"). And that was only on the first day that they took speed. By the third day of speed use, the subjects had numerous negative things to say ("a bad drug effect," "dizzy," and "flu-like symptoms"). Poor sleep and poor appetite may have been in part responsible. Taking amphetamines orally, even the most potent one, methamphetamine, does not produce a sustained high. Amphetamines have to be inhaled or injected to produce a high; that's the only way they reach the brain quickly.

Your child may be affected by other childrens' interest in obtaining stimulants. A survey of 14,000 high school students revealed that 5% took stimulants for ADHD. Of that group, 15% reported having given some of their medication to others, 7% had sold some of their medication, 4% had experienced theft of their medication, and 3% had "been forced" to give up some of their medication. Stimulant abuse was related to access: the more children at a school who were receiving stimulants for ADHD, the more students there were who abused them. However, we can not stop giving stimulants to children who need them just because they can be abused. Conversely, we do have to monitor carefully to minimize this problem. You can help your children to handle the peer pressure by teaching them to just say no, and by reporting efforts at coercion to school authorities (many schools already require that medication be dispersed by the school nurse, eliminating that hazard, at least on school grounds). Besides that, your children can use the excuse that their doctor or parent counts their pills. Every state tracks the number of prescriptions written for stimulants by various practitioners and for whom the prescription is written in a central location. In some states, doctors are legally bound to notify police if they discover the prescription is being misused.

59. How do I know the right time to start giving my child ADHD medication? And how long will my child need to stay on stimulants?

In younger children, a teacher is generally going to be the one to let you know. If you receive phone calls from someone at the school or feel pressured at parent–teacher conference, it is time to think seriously about medication. A teacher's comments about your child being hyperactive, impulsive, easily distracted, or inattentive are worth discussing with your pediatrician or other medical specialists. This may also be the time to get a more formal evaluation, either through the school system or independently through a private psychologist. It could take the form of standardized questionnaires about attention or a formal neuropsychological evaluation to assess IQ, academics, and emotional status.

In dealing with older children who have over the years managed to handle their ADHD-related difficulties, you should consider the possibility of ADHD treatment if their grades begin to drop, their homework is regularly missing, they are increasingly disorganized, and/or their school work begins to take an unreasonable amount of time. Again, it's worth discussing the situation with their teacher and your pediatrician or other physician specialists. This is the time to get an evaluation.

If the diagnosis is uncertain, the decision about taking medication can sometimes be even harder. As no biological marker for ADHD exists at this time, at some level the diagnosis is always probable rather than absolute. Sometimes, the discussion about medication treatment hinges on whether giving medication to a child who does not have true ADHD is worse than withholding medication from one who really does. Stimulant medications (discussed in Questions 45–48) work very quickly. Thus, you can generally figure out within a week or two whether medication is working. Because you will have your answer very quickly, no harm is done by trying medication. If the medication helps, the response is dramatic. Generally, your reservations will disappear just as fast.

You do not have to make the decision about using medication on the spot. The professional discussing medication with you will talk about the pros and cons. Then you should go home and read. Plenty of books and Internet resources (discussed in the Appendix) can enlighten you about ADHD. Talk it over with your spouse and family; include your child if he or she is old enough to consider the options.

Although teachers and other school officials may suggest that your child take medication, they cannot prescribe it or force it on your child. Strict laws govern the prescription of stimulants. Some school systems also have guidelines for the appropriate level of school involvement. However, do not assume that teachers—if they are the ones who suggest medication—just want a quiet, compliant child in the classroom. They more than likely have your child's best interests at heart.

If you do choose to use medication, you should notify the school. School personnel need to know about any medication your child is taking so they can deal properly with any emergency health issues. Medication management is also part of a complete package you should develop with the school to optimize your ADHD child's education.

Wondering how long your child will need to take medication is a common question. Sometimes it's asked even before a decision about using medication is made. People used to think that most children outgrew their ADHD around puberty, but studies now show that this is not true. In many children, ADHD persists indefinitely (discussed in Question 98), although it may take different forms, and treatment strategies may change. The duration of treatment varies, with some children requiring treatment into and throughout adulthood. No crystal ball answer exists; only time provides a way to figure this out. Each academic and life milestone produces new challenges, and you need to reassess the necessity for medication continually. If you are considering discontinuing medication, it is generally best to start the school year on medication and then stop in October or November. This way your child's performance on and off medication can be compared.

If you are considering discontinuing medication, it is generally best to start the school year on medication and then stop in October or November.

Going to college is not easy for anyone. Many ADHD teenagers succeed in high school in part because of parental support. Parents watch over their homework, get them to doctor's appointments, and make sure that their medication prescriptions are refilled. When teenagers go to college, their support systems disappear abruptly. Students may receive some support from the disability office at the college, but this help does not substitute for a parent. In fact, many ADHD students fear some stigma and shy away from using the disability office when they first arrive at college, the time when they probably need it most. College students with ADHD may run into new difficulties when they have to regulate their own life. Getting enough sleep may prove to be a problem. Also, they may have trouble getting up in time for class with no one there to wake them or make sure that they stay awake when the alarm clock sounds.

Physicians ought to provide as much structure as possible for ADHD adolescents who are leaving home for college or independent living. Doctors have to help plan how prescriptions are going to be refilled, where medications will be kept, and how to ensure that medications are taken regularly. College students may find that carrying medications in a backpack can be useful in that it allows them take a pill during class if they have forgotten to take it earlier. If it is on hand, they can take it on the spot.

Teenagers often want to discontinue their medications when they leave home. Obviously, the decision is ultimately up to them. However, this decision should be made in consultation with their treating physician. If these youngsters have a long-term relationship with their doctor, an office consultation prior to going off to college is a definite benefit. Going to college with medication and getting started on the right foot is generally the best strategy. Perhaps in October or November such students can reconsider whether continuing medication is necessary. If they discontinue medication, they ought to reevaluate their performance in college shortly thereafter to make sure that they continue to succeed. This strategy provides for personal control but also is scientific and makes good sense. Getting adolescents back to their treating physician may be difficult after they have gone off to college, but it is a particularly important time to monitor their performance and regulate medications appropriately. They ought to schedule vacation visits well in advance.

The use of alcohol and recreational drugs can cause problems for high school and college students with ADHD. They may want to stop their medication because they do not know how it will interact with these substances, and students who do not have ADHD may ask them to share their stimulant medications. Parents must discuss these issues with all ADHD students before they leave for college. Stimulants can have an additive effect with alcohol and recreational drugs. Thus, stimulant medications should not be taken at the same time as alcohol and recreational drugs. Fortunately, most alcohol and recreational drugs are used in the evening when stimulant effects should have waned. A frank discussion with a doctor about medication interactions is the best tactic. Doctors should instruct ADHD students not to give away any of their medications. They may blame this on the doctor—"He counts my pills"—as a face-saving response. The doctor should also instruct them to keep their medications in a safe place where other students will not find them. Sometimes, counting pills is actually necessary for teenagers to make sure that they're not giving medications to other students or using more medications than they should.

Stimulants can have an additive effect with alcohol and recreational drugs. Thus, stimulant medications should not be taken at the same time as alcohol and recreational drugs.

60. Must I make regular visits to the doctor, or can medications be adjusted by phone?

Your doctor often finds things out at a visit that could be missed in a phone conversation. After all, as a parent you do not always know what's important and what isn't. This is highlighted by the MTA study (see Question 46). The medication group managed by the experts fared significantly better than did the routine community care group, even though these children also received medication. Some people adjust to medication better than others. The study experts took special care during the first month of treatment to find an optimal dose of medication for each child. Thereafter, they saw children monthly for half-hour visits. During the visits, the prescribing doctor spoke with the parent, met with the child, and discussed any concerns that the family might have regarding the medication or the child's ADHD-related difficulties. If the child was experiencing any difficulties, the MTA physician-expert considered adjustments in the child's medication rather than taking a "wait-and-see" approach. MTA physicians prescribed doses (the MTA study was performed with short-acting medications) that were higher and more frequent than those used by the community physicians because they took a more forceful approach to weighing the effectiveness of treatment. Also, the MTA physician-expert was in contact with the school. Sometimes, even though a parent is not getting calls from individuals at school, school issues remain. Medication dose adjustment may solve these more minor school issues. The goal in the MTA study was to adjust medication to a point that left "no room for improvement." Close supervision also permitted early detection and response to any problematic side effects from medication, a process that may have improved efforts to help children to continue effective treatment. Finally, although the physicians in the MTA medication-only group did not provide behavioral therapy, they did advise involved parents about any problems their child may have been experiencing and provided reading materials and additional information as requested. By contrast, visits to community doctors checking on medication occurred on average every 6 months and lasted about 15 minutes each. The doctors did not contact anyone at the school. A wait-and-see attitude was common.

61. Does my child have to take stimulant medication every day, or are drug holidays possible?

Whether your child should take medication for 365 days a year, on school days only, for summer camp, or for sports depends on individual needs and schedule. Some children find that their ADHD is troublesome only when they are performing academic tasks and that they can do without medication on weekends, on school holidays, or during the summer. Others can not do this and, therefore, require daily medication. Remember: ADHD can affect function both in and away from school. Functioning adequately is not the same thing as getting the most out of time at the museum, the playground, the movies, a play date, or summer camp. ADHD children should take medication when it's needed. Don't skimp!

Remember: ADHD can affect function both in and away from school.

Some children need medication only on school days because lack of focus and attention interferes significantly with schoolwork only. Nevertheless, learning takes place all the time, not only during the school day. Most children who need medication in school need it when doing homework as well. Studies show that medication enhances both children's learning and practicing what they learn while medicated (e.g., doing homework). This means that going to school and doing homework while taking medication are better than taking medication only while at school. Learning is better consolidated when the brain is in the "same biochemical state." The concept of "same-state" learning can also be applied to weekends. Sometimes, using a lower dose on weekends or timing medication with weekend study time turns out to be a good compromise.

Deciding whether to use medication on weekends as a way of treating ADHD behaviors can be a tough one. Because the decision is a very individual choice, often no right or wrong answer exists. Weekend time is usually more parent–child oriented, and many parents can manage their ADHD children on weekends without medication. However, the question remains: What price will you pay? If you're constantly disciplining your child, no one's having any fun, and your child's self esteem may suffer. Medication has been shown to enhance parenting skills. The parents of children who take medication are better able to deal with their children. They do not need to be as controlling and can use more positive backup. If discipline is the issue, you ought at least to carefully consider using medication on the weekends. Children with the hyperactive–impulsive and the combined types of ADHD are particularly likely to need medication every day, as are children with associated conduct disorders. Medication is helpful in minimizing their impulsivity and thereby improving their social interactions with family and friends (discussed in Question 55). Conversely, inattentive children may not obviously suffer without medication on the weekend, unless they have homework to complete. However, one can again make the argument that inattentive children miss social cues without medication and gain less from family activities.

Sometimes a child's age plays a role in deciding whether to use medication on non-school days. Parents are often good reporters about the daily behavior of pre-school and elementary school-age children. Conversely, they may not be as aware of the problems that a teenager is having during evenings and weekends. A teenager's weekend problems can involve organizing and planning long-term projects for school, but they can also reflect difficulties in coping with complex social situations (e.g., decisions about drug and alcohol use). Medication may enhance self-control and decrease impulsivity. This is also true for driving, in which less impulsivity and improved attention may decrease the risk of accidents (discussed in Question 97). One recent study using a simulated driving setup documented a correlation between improved driving performance and long-acting medication, thus highlighting the advantages of continuous medication for facing the demands of everyday life.

Questions about whether to use stimulant medication at summer camp are common. Some children, particularly those with hyperactive–impulsive or combined type ADHD or those whose social skills are helped by medication, ought to take medication during summer camp even though the activities at summer camp may help them to expend some or even most of their excess energy. Other children do fine without medication.

Drug holidays typically coincide with school holidays and vacation. ADHD children who are more likely to take "drug holidays" include older, less affected children; those with the inattention subtype; and those who have fewer hyperactivity–impulsivity symptoms at baseline. Research, however, shows that many parents' satisfaction ratings (how they felt about family) dip during drug holidays. Drug holidays are certainly not mandatory and may not be a plus.

No medical concern argues against daily stimulant medication. No studies show more side effects when medicine is used every day as opposed to only weekdays. Unless your child has significant problems with eating when using stimulant medication, you ought to consider carefully a decision against everyday medication. After all, once you've decided that medicine is acceptable and you see it working for your child, "less is not necessarily more." Children with ADHD should take medications to cover times at which they have problems. Although parents' continuing concerns about the effects of medication often lead them to want to minimize the times at which their children take medications, the best choice is to medicate children during times when their ADHD symptoms interfere with their everyday life. Under-treating children who are having problems during weekends, vacations, or summers has no long-term advantages. Indeed, it may have long-term disadvantages. However, some children definitely need medicine only from Monday through Friday during the school year.

62. My teenager's medication has been working well throughout his high school years. Do we need to consider other factors and make changes in his medication before he heads off to college?

As a general rule, most college students do not get up at 7:00 AM for classes. They also may take naps in the middle of the day or stay up late into the wee hours of the morning to study. Although long-acting medication might have been used throughout high school, some college students prefer short-acting medication which they can tailor to their own needs. It is very important that, prior to going to college, you and your child work with your physician to develop a medication plan that is realistic for your college student. This medication plan should include not only which medication should be prescribed, but also how the student will remember to take the medication and how it will be renewed.

The way your child obtains medication while he or she is at college needs to be planned. Does he go directly to a doctor at home or at college? Does he receive his medication through his parents? Once your child gets to college, there are alternative ways of proceeding. After the student settles in and finds out his schedule, he can get in touch with the hometown physician, either by phone or email. As your adolescent is now an adult, it most certainly becomes his responsibility to make regular contact with the physician. If you are obtaining the medication from the pharmacy, have a designated plan with your child. Get an idea about when in each calendar month the renewal is due. For example, plan to renew the first week of each month, so the medication will reach your student by the second week.

A second alternative is to work with the hometown physician or the school to find a new psychiatrist or neurologist at the college or in the surrounding community who will monitor and prescribe your child's medication. Because these medications are controlled substances, out-of-state prescriptions may not be honored. Rather than mailing medication from home, it is also possible that your student can obtain it directly from a pharmacy on or close to campus. This decision may depend on your insurance coverage and where your child attends school.

It is very important that, prior to going to college, you and your child work with your physician to develop a medication plan that is realistic for your college student.

Medication and ADHD

63. My son is going off to college. I am even more worried about abuse. Should I be?

There are several abuse issues that your child may run into in college. For one, college students are now in control of their own medication. This makes them vulnerable to internal or external pressures. Selling stimulants is illegal, but it does occur at college. Other students may want medication, not just to get high but to get work done. You and your doctor need to talk with your child about this before he heads off to college. Discussion should focus on how to say "no" and strategies about how to keep medication in a private and secure place. In addition, another topic of discussion should be about how much your child wants to let his peers know about his diagnosis or use of medication.

Abuse comes in many forms. When used properly, an individual cannot get high on ADHD medication. However, if stimulant medications are ground up and subsequently, snorted or taken intravenously, they can make someone high. Other students may try to buy or steal your teenager's medication for this purpose.

Another way some students abuse their medications is by taking too much of it. They falsely believe that more medication will enhance their power of concentration and improve their performance. Too much medicine will probably make your child jittery and actually be counter-productive in terms of getting work accomplished. Using too much medicine for long periods of time can be dangerous, so parents and physicians need to be on the lookout. Sometimes too high a dose turns out to be a way of self medicating depression.

One recent study looked at misuse by college students. Few college students with a prescription for ADHD medication took their medication other than as prescribed, by taking it at higher doses or at greater frequency. Although this is concerning, it is important to recognize that most students who misused their ADHD medication did so only to try to improve their academic performance. This kind of misuse suggests that many students find their treatment to be less helpful than they would like. Physicians who treat college students with ADHD need to take late night symptom coverage into account in their prescribing regime. But they also need to minimize potential adverse effects on sleep.

Several aspects of students' misuse are particularly concerning. Nearly 8% of the students in the study reported that they had snorted their medication in the past 6 months, nearly 30% had used it in conjunction with alcohol, and 20% had used along with marijuana; these behaviors have potentially negative health consequences that students may not fully understand.

Another concern was that 25% of students had given medication to a friend and most had been asked to. Physicians need to discuss medication diversion with college students and to contract with them about not diverting their medication. Of course, carefully monitoring what students are doing with their medications is extremely difficult, particularly when prescribing physicians may often be located in students' hometowns rather than where they attend school.

Charles's comment:

My son Bob told me that he was frequently asked to sell his medication to other students. We talked a lot about the difficult position that this put him in. He practiced answers and learned ways to say "no," responding that he was going to earn far more money in the long run taking his medication and doing better in school than selling medication for imme-diate cash.

64. Do the type or differing symptoms of ADHD affect treatment choices?

The MTA stimulant study, described in Question 46, found no difference in decrease of core ADHD symptoms (hyperactivity, inattention, impulsivity) between those in the group who were expertly medicated and given behavioral therapy and those in the group who were expertly medicated only. However, in other areas of functioning—specifically, anxiety symptoms, academics, conduct disorder and oppositional behavior, parent–child relations, and teacher-rated social skills— the combined treatment approach was better. In addition, those in the combined-treatment group needed lower doses of medication as compared to those in the researcher-treated medication-only group.

Children who have a comorbid disorder sometimes require two medications.

The presence of comorbid disorders also affects how well stimulants work. Although the rule of thumb is to treat the primary ADHD disorder first, children who have a comorbid disorder sometimes require two medications. For example, a doctor might use both a stimulant and an antidepressant to treat a child with ADHD and depression, or he might use both a stimulant and clonidine to treat a child with a conduct disorder. Children with co-occurring intellectual disability and autistic spectrum disorders (see Questions 43 and 44) may be more sensitive to medication, require lower doses, and potentially have more side effects.

Different doses of stimulant medication have different effects on ADHD symptoms. Medication often has its first effect on behavior. Only over time, and sometimes with increased dosage, does it have an effect on attention.

In other words, lower doses of medicine improve behavior, and higher doses are often needed to really enhance attention. Thus, your doctor must carefully adjust medication dosages. You should not necessarily maintain the dose that results in improved behavior. Teacher input about behavior in class and academic performance can optimize treatment.

THE NONSTIMULANTS

65. What are the other medications for ADHD? What are the pros and cons of nonstimulant medication?

The stimulants are very likely to be effective in most children with ADHD and, because they pass in and out of the system quickly, we also can determine their effectiveness quickly (1 to 2 weeks). None of the nonstimulant medications have the same likelihood of effectiveness as that of the stimulant medications, and all require daily administration to maintain a therapeutic level in the body. (Of course, if they work for your child, the effectiveness issue becomes moot.) However, in children who can not handle stimulants, find stimulants not fully effective, or have particular comorbid disorders, other medications may be useful alone or in combination with stimulants. Other medications probably work because they affect the same neurotransmitters (discussed in Question 8) as those affected by the stimulants, although to different degrees.

The **selective serotonin reuptake inhibitors (SSRIs)** were originally developed to treat depression. Prozac is the prototype. Other SSRIs, the brand names of which you may recognize, are Zoloft, Paxil, Celexa, Lexapro, and Luvox. The latter is particularly good for treating

Medication and ADHD

None of the nonstimulant medications have the same likelihood of effectiveness as that of the stimulant medications, and all require daily administration to maintain a therapeutic level in the body.

Selective serotonin reuptake inhibitors (SSRIs)

Medications that work by inhibiting the serotonin transporter. Therefore serotonin, which would ordinarily be shuttled into the neuron, remains in the synapse for a longer period of time, until it diffuses away or is destroyed by an enzyme.

obsessive-compulsive disorder (a disorder that can occur with ADHD and is discussed in Question 39).

Not only do the SSRIs have an antidepressant effect, they tend to diminish anxiety. Both depression and anxiety can accompany ADHD. Thus, doctors might use an SSRI along with a stimulant in children with comorbid anxiety and depression. Some studies have shown that an SSRI may help ADHD directly. Doctors should choose medication to treat the primary problem first. SSRIs sometime smooth the effect of the stimulants over the day, minimizing its ups and downs. They may also minimize the flatness of a child who is otherwise responding well to stimulants, thereby allowing for continuing use and benefit.

Side effects of SSRIs include the usual: headache, nausea, sleep disturbances, change in appetite, and dry mouth. However, these effects are generally very mild or transient, if they occur at all, and they rarely limit treatment. Impotence and decreased libido are not issues for children, although if such effects occur, adolescents could find them problematic. SSRIs must be taken daily to be effective. Deciding whether the SSRIs and the other antidepressants are effective can take several weeks.

The press has focused a lot of attention recently on the possibility that Paxil and other SSRIs may increase the risk of suicide in children and that it may produce problematic side effects when stopped. These caveats should not prohibit choosing an SSRI, but Paxil and the other SSRIs should be tapered slowly, and any child treated for depression should be carefully monitored.

The three atypical antidepressants that have been used to treat ADHD are Wellbutrin, Cymbalta, and Effexor.

Some studies have shown that Wellbutrin can treat ADHD. It may also work synergistically with the stimulants, enhancing their effectiveness. Again, if comorbid depression is present, Wellbutrin could be considered. Wellbutrin in lower doses contains the same ingredient as that in the medications used to help smokers to stop smoking. Because Wellbutrin increases norepinephrine (the main frontal lobe neurotransmitter) as well as dopamine, it may improve motivation. The more common side effects are agitation, confusion, headache, nausea, vomiting, sleep disturbances, change in appetite, and dry mouth. Some studies have also shown that Effexor or Cymbalta can improve ADHD symptoms. These medications are serotonin and norepinephrine reuptake inhibitors (SNRIs). They increase both norepinephrine and serotonin levels. Again, if comorbid depression is present, your doctor could consider Effexor or Cymbalta. The more common side effects are agitation, headache, nausea, insomnia, change in appetite, sweating, and dry mouth.

In **clinical trials** during the 1980s, researchers evaluated the effectiveness of the tricyclic antidepressant drugs, such as Tofranil (a medication that once was commonly used for nighttime bedwetting), and Elavil in children with ADHD. The tricyclics may initially be as effective as the stimulant drugs, but their effectiveness was not sustained. Now that we have more choices of medications, tricyclics are used less often because of their relatively lesser effectiveness and their side effects. Doctors now use Desipramine most often in treating adolescents with coexisting tics, those with tics occasionally worsened by stimulants, and in some who do not respond to stimulants. Because newer antidepressants like the SSRIs and the SNRIs have fewer side effects, the tricyclics are generally not a first choice

Clinical trial

A carefully monitored study of a drug or a treatment using a drug that involves a large group of people with the goal of testing that drug's effectiveness.

Because newer antidepressants like the SSRIs and the SNRIs have fewer side effects, the tricyclics are generally not a first choice for children with comorbid depression.

for children with comorbid depression. The advantages of the tricyclic antidepressant medications include their relatively long **half-life** (which means that children do not have to take them during school hours), slower waning of action, and minimal risk of abuse.

Half-life

A measure of the duration of a drug's action, how long it takes before one-half the dose is gone. Drugs with long half-lives can be given infrequently, whereas drugs with short half-lives need to be given frequently.

Tricyclic antidepressants need to be taken daily. They can cause dry mouth, and in some children they have proved to be sedating and to cause unacceptable fatigue. Conversely, in ADHD children with sleep problems, they may have a beneficial effect at bedtime. Cardiac side effects have proved to be the most serious; several otherwise healthy ADHD children treated with tricyclics (ages 5 to 14 years) died suddenly. However, considering the long years of Tofranil usage for bedwetting without incident, it seems likely that these most unfortunate events fall within the range of sudden unexplained death in childhood. Since routine monitoring of blood drug levels and electrocardiograms do not predict these catastrophic events, doctors recommend the tricyclics in children only if stimulant drugs prove ineffective and if coexisting disorders (e.g., depression or tics) interfere seriously with normal functioning. Periodic blood levels and follow-up electrocardiograms are appropriate. Newer antidepressants in the SSRI family are probably a better choice for most children with ADHD and comorbid depression.

66. What are clonidine and guanfacine/ Tenex, and what are their side effects?

Both clonidine (Catapres) and guanfacine (Tenex) are partial agonist drugs that increase norepinephrine release, especially in the frontal lobe, and have been found to be effective for treating children with ADHD, with tics, and with ADHD and tics. Researchers originally developed them to treat hypertension. They tend to be more effective for hyperactivity and conduct problems than for attention. Overall, they are not as effective as the stimulant medications. However, one recent study of children with ADHD and tics found that combined clonidine and Ritalin was more effective than Ritalin alone for treating ADHD.

For some children, clonidine has proved to be sedating and cause unacceptable fatigue. Sometimes, this side effect can be put to good use by helping a child fall asleep after a small dose at bedtime. On occasion, clonidine makes children irritable. Tenex tends to be less sedating and has a longer half-life, which means it lasts longer. Thus, while ADHD children must take both clonidine and Tenex daily, they can use Tenex less frequently (once or twice a day versus two to three times a day). A new once-a-day long-acting form of guanfacine (Intuniv) has just been released. Clonidine comes in the form of a patch that continuously releases the medication and is changed once a week. The advantage is obvious.

Cardiac issues are the most serious potential side effect of both clonidine and Tenex. A few reports of sudden unexplained death in children taking both stimulants and clonidine have raised questions about the cardiac safety of the stimulants and clonidine–Tenex in combination. The individuals reported had not been screened for subclinical cardiac problems prior to treatment. They were all taking other medications as well. Researchers have conducted controlled clinical trials using combined stimulants and clonidine in children with tics and ADHD without incident. The frequency of documented sudden death is considered to be within the range of that which can be anticipated in childhood—extraordinarily rare, but possible.

67. What about Strattera? How well does it work and what are its side effects?

Strattera has proven to be quite effective for treating ADHD and has a mechanism of action that differs from that of the stimulants. In contrast to the stimulants, which primarily affect dopamine, Strattera is a norepinephrine reuptake inhibitor, thus it increases brain norepinephrine levels (discussed in Question 8). The precise role that norepinephrine plays in ADHD is not known. However, scientists believe it may be important in regulating attention, impulsivity, and activity levels. In all the clinical trials, Strattera was superior to placebo in reducing the symptoms of ADHD in children, adolescents, and adults. Strattera produced positive effects on all ADHD symptoms, including hyperactivity– impulsiveness and inattention. Adolescents and younger children with ADHD get similar benefits from Strattera despite age-related differences in symptoms.

Strattera needs to be taken every day to maintain a steady-state blood level. It also takes time to build up in your body. Adjusting the dose and deciding whether Strattera is effective may take as long as a month or more. This medication seems to be particularly useful in treating children who become anxious on stimulant medications. Many physicians are starting to use stimulants and Strattera in combination. The Strattera allows for lower doses of stimulant medications, minimizing stimulant side effects. Strattera could be especially useful for families with ADHD children who have difficulty with the transitions of getting their children to bed at night and waking them up in the morning. Strattera may also turn out to be especially useful for children with ADHD and tics, as it shares some biochemical effects in common with clonidine–Tenex, both recommended anti-tic medicines.

Some children may lose weight when starting treatment with Strattera. As with all ADHD medications, a doctor should monitor their growth during treatment. In clinical studies, most children who experienced side effects were not bothered enough to stop using Strattera. The most common side effects were upset stomach, decreased appetite, nausea and vomiting, dizziness, tiredness, and mood swings. Generally, these side effects were temporary. Strattera is metabolized in your liver. Because of its particular pattern of metabolism, it interacts with some other commonly used medications. These include some of the selective serotonin reuptake inhibitors (SSRIs; discussed in Question 65) and some asthma medicines. Although this does not mean that you can not take Strattera with any other medications, your doctor has to be particularly careful about adjusting the dosages. Your doctor will probably check your child's liver function periodically, since on rare occasions Strattera can affect the liver.

68. Are other options besides traditional medications useful for treating ADHD? Can behavioral modification be used in lieu of stimulant medication? Are nonmedicinal remedies, such as vitamins or dietary changes, useful for treating ADHD?

Studies clearly show that properly used medication is by far the most effective therapy for ADHD. For example, the MTA study showed that medication monitored by experts was significantly more effective than intensive behavioral therapy. The behavioral therapy evaluated in the MTA study (Question 46) consisted of 2 months of an immersion summer camp program; 12 weeks of somebody coming to the school every day

Studies clearly show that properly used medication is by far the most effective therapy for ADHD.

to work with the teachers; 26 weeks of parent training, so the parents could use these techniques at home; and 26 weeks of individual and group therapy. In other words, it was a very money- , labor- , and time-intensive treatment. Medication worked better for the core symptoms of ADHD—hyperactivity, impulsivity, and inattention.

A number of dietary supplements, including megavitamins, minerals, and St. John's wort, have been touted to help in treating ADHD symptoms. Scientific studies do not support the claim. Beware: What you buy in an herbal food store is generally untested and is not necessarily safe. Some commonly used herbs and high doses of ordinarily safe foods or vitamin supplements can interact with prescription medications and alter their effect.

Dietary restrictions have long been hailed as a way of treating ADHD. The Feingold diet was popular in the 1970s, but lacked proof that it ever worked, and it wreaked havoc in the kitchen for everyone. With this diet, you could not eat such foods as apples or tomatoes. No scientific evidence supports the claim that sugar makes children hyperactive, even though many people think so. Sugar is, of course, fattening and can cause cavities. For those reasons, we should eat it in moderation. Food additives and preservatives have a bad name, but no scientific data really prove that they are bad for you. Of course, eating a healthy, well-balanced diet is a good idea for all children.

PART FOUR

Negotiating for Academic Success

What kinds of learning difficulties are commonly associated with ADHD?

What accommodations should I encourage the school to make for my ADHD child?

What is an IEP, and why do ADHD students need one?

More . . .

69. What kinds of learning difficulties are commonly associated with ADHD?

According to the statistics, some 50% of ADHD children have learning disabilities. It is important to remember that ADHD by itself is not officially classified as a learning disorder; however, with increasing frequency, schools are recognizing many of the learning problems that are commonly associated with ADHD. Although the attention-related problems themselves do not meet standards for a classifiable learning disability, these learning issues may significantly interfere with success in children's academic life. For example, children with ADHD may have difficulties with learning rote information. Not only are these children not always listening when the information is presented, but they also have more trouble retaining material that is not presented in a contextual or meaningful way. This may cause problems in various subject areas, such as learning history dates, foreign language vocabulary, or math facts. Such children may also require additional time for taking classroom and standardized tests because their vulnerability to distractibility interferes with their rapid processing of information.

The literature indicates that children who are inattentive, overly active, impulsive, and easily distracted commonly experience poor academic performance. Typical problem areas for ADHD children (e.g., procrastination, trouble with planning and organizing, difficulty retaining learned material and in interactions with others) can most certainly create learning problems that apply to any subject matter. Inconsistent performance is also a common complaint of parents with ADHD children. Furthermore, findings suggest that children with ADHD perform more poorly than do other children on standardized measures of achievement.

There is a high probability that children with ADHD may have comorbid learning problems. In fact, research indicates that approximately 20% to 25% of children with ADHD have a comorbid learning disability. Conversely, about 15% of those children with learning disabilities also have ADHD. Children who fail to develop specific academic abilities by a proper age or grade level relative to their intellectual capacities are considered to have learning disabilities. A number of different learning disorders are seen in ADHD children. They include reading disabilities, mathematics disabilities, disorders of written expression, specific receptive and expressive language problems, and coordination difficulties that can affect both gross and fine motor skills, including handwriting.

Research indicates that approximately 20% to 25% of children with ADHD have a comorbid learning disability.

Interestingly, a group of Scandinavian psychiatrists have coined the acronym "DAMP" to describe a complex of symptoms seen in ADHD children: disorders of attention, motor functioning, and visual-spatial perception. In addition, some children with ADHD have nonverbal learning disabilities (NVLD). Children with such disabilities can have prominent visual-spatial and/or visual-motor difficulties, executive planning problems, sensory and motor problems, and social skill difficulties. For these children, academic problems show up mainly in mathematics, science, written expression, and reading comprehension, particularly as the child advances in school. However, in order to determine whether or not a child has learning issues associated with ADHD or a learning disorder comorbidly accompanying a diagnosis of ADHD, a thorough assessment of a child's skills is recommended (see Question 32).

70. Will some school subjects or activities be more difficult for my ADHD child?

Yes. Certain areas of a standard school curriculum tend to be more difficult for ADHD children. For example,

ADHD children frequently have difficulties with listening well and/or rote memorization. Therefore, classes that put more emphasis on oral presentation and retaining facts may be more problematic. Many ADHD children have trouble learning foreign languages. Their attention strays when so much verbal material is presented. They also struggle with the routine repetition necessary to learn vocabulary words. Similarly, the rote memorization required for mathematics may be difficult. Whether it involves learning addition or subtraction facts, memorizing geometry theorems, or recalling the multiplication tables, mathematics class can be a problem. A good performance in such a class also requires a systematic, organized approach to a task. ADHD students commonly hand in messy papers. They often have problems organizing their work on the written page and struggle to follow a step-by-step approach to a task. They may also miss important math signs (i.e., a plus or a minus), making errors that are due to their inattentiveness, not to their ability.

In general, ADHD students perform best in classes that maintain a hands-on approach, break up learning into small chunks, and encourage class participation. Teacher style is also very important, as classes that are comprised of long lectures or darkened auditoriums for slide presentations may not be optimal for an ADHD child. Classes that focus on long-term projects may also be problematic unless the student's progress is supported by ongoing monitoring.

71. Does having ADHD make reading difficult for my child?

Although ADHD does not cause a reading disability or dyslexia, it definitely can have effects on reading performance. In other words, children with ADHD do not necessarily have problems with decoding, the sounding out of words. However, ADHD children can have difficulties in accurately and efficiently tracking down a page or staying focused when reading long passages. ADHD children may score poorly on standardized tests of reading when they are required to sit quietly for extended lengths of time in a large group, silently read several long passages, and answer multiple-choice questions. They may also have trouble switching back and forth between questions and separate answer sheets. Thus, the problem may not be their weak decoding or impaired reading comprehension. In essence, their limited capacity to sustain focus or attend to details masquerades as a reading problem. It is very important to remember that ADHD and dyslexia are two different disorders. Having both ADHD and dyslexia, however, can be particularly problematic, as the lack of sustained focus and distractibility can make the process of learning to read even more difficult.

Donna's comment:

Jeffrey was placed in "Reading Recovery" at school. As bright as he was, he needed remedial reading! I went to observe him and saw that he could not sit still long enough to learn to read! I called the doctor that same day.

72. I know that disorganization is my child's biggest problem. What can I do to help?

This is an area in which parents can be quite helpful. At the beginning of each school year, parents can assist students in their efforts to organize their binders and other school materials. Develop a system that is easy and efficient and makes your child comfortable. For example, your child can use several large binders with color-coding to identify sectioned-off areas for individual subjects. In addition, separate sections for assignments or completed homework might be useful. Most students also need to have a means to coordinate and flag after-school activities, homework, and long-term projects. A portable visual aid, such as a calendar or day-timer, is another important tool that can help organize a student's time and activities. In addition, some children may do better with a visual system, such as a large wall or desk calendar, at their workspace.

Since the workspace itself can be a huge source of inefficiency, it is a place to focus parental attention. First, ADHD children need a routine place to work where distractions are minimal and all the necessary supplies are close at hand. Although most ADHD children require a homework setting with limited distractions, some may possibly work better with background music. Essentially, the music serves to help these students stay on task. Also, working in a quiet setting does not mean that the student should be "out of contact" with the rest of the family. There are times when these children may not be making noise, but they may also not be doing their homework. A workspace should be accessible to routine surprise visits by parents.

Parents should work with their children to design, supply, and organize the workspace. An appropriate workspace means an area that includes both a computer and space to perform handwritten assignments. Pencils, erasers, paper clips, a stapler, and the like should all be readily available. Teenagers most certainly will request accessible connections to the Internet and telephone; however, be aware that those technological advances bring their own distractions.

73. My child hates doing homework and procrastinates all the time. What strategies can help us to get through each evening?

Households with ADHD children must develop homework routines. Such routines should encompass when and where the work must be done. For example, homework may be done right after school or right after dinner. Whatever works for a particular child and family is perfectly fine as long as both agree to establish and maintain the routine. Parents should limit distractions and state clear expectations. Obviously, with ADHD children, rules and follow-through are particularly important. For example, when it is determined that there is no television watching until work is completed, parents must enforce the rule.

ADHD children also require frequent "study breaks." Therefore, it is important to agree upon an appropriate amount of time in which the student can maintain attention before a break is needed. Setting a kitchen timer is a good method for making this point visible and concrete to a child. A specific reward system can also be helpful. In that way, students can earn snacks or the privilege of watching a television program when they stay on task with their work.

Your participation in your child's homework routine on a daily basis is crucial. ADHD children take much longer than might be expected to reach a point at which they can work alone. They may need you to sit with them each and every night, not just to help with problems or projects but simply to be there in the room. In fact, a parent's physical presence is a vital factor. Sometimes parents become frustrated with an ADHD child's inability to work independently. No doubt the homework process can be very time demanding, particularly

ADHD children take much longer than might be expected to reach a point at which they can work alone.

after an adult's long day. Yet, parents need to remember that ADHD children need their active support until they have successfully mastered the skills necessary for them to work on their own, and that can take many years.

In many households, parents can and do provide the necessary academic support. Particularly during the elementary school years, parents need to spend the evening time setting priorities for assignments, organizing materials, clarifying instructions, or answering questions. Nevertheless, as the work becomes more complex and the child's demands for independence increase, it may become more difficult for parents to successfully "tutor" their own children. Then, parents are encouraged to look for one of several types of homework support. Sometimes a homework helper can be a good choice. In those instances, the ADHD child may require only the physical presence of an older adolescent or young adult to reinforce motivation, provide organizational support, and answer general questions. If junior high and high school students need help in a particular subject area, a subject tutor may be a more appropriate solution. Many ADHD children, however, require more general homework support. Sometimes, an organizational tutor can be the most beneficial in teaching the important study strategies that are a key to success across a variety of subject areas.

74. My child is fascinated with basketball. Will ADHD make team sports participation impossible?

ADHD most certainly does not make participating in team sports impossible for students; however, it may make it more difficult. ADHD children can be wonderful athletes. Many famous athletes are testimony to that fact. Nevertheless, difficulties can arise for ADHD children when they are playing team sports. They may have trouble following complex instructions, multitasking, or responding cooperatively to authority. Some ADHD students favor individualized sports, such as tennis or golf, rather than the more traditional team sports, such as soccer or basketball. Either way, athletics and team sports can be an area in which ADHD students receive positive feedback and increase self-esteem. It may be helpful, however, to have a discussion with the coach in order to provide information about the best ways to instruct your child. Another issue to consider is medication. In other words, if medication is necessary during school hours in order to increase concentration and focus, is medication also needed when your child plays sports after school? If so, it will be necessary to work out the dose, the time, and the manner in which the medication will be administered.

75. Can my ADHD child be successful in a mainstream classroom?

Yes, your child quite possibly—and actually very probably—can be successful in mainstream education. However, there is a growing awareness in the education community that ADHD can cause significant learning problems for children. For these ADHD children, specific accommodations may improve their chance of success. These arrangements may vary, depending on your child's specific needs, and can range from such things as extended time for taking tests to tape recording lectures. Another smaller group of ADHD children may do better in special education classrooms where there are lower student-to-teacher ratios, where the setting is extremely structured, and where the expectations are very clear. Special education placement may also relate to whether your ADHD child has other comorbid conditions, such as learning disabilities or psychiatric problems, which require intensive academic or emotional support.

76. Should I inform the teachers that my child has ADHD?

Absolutely. Taking a proactive stance in your child's education is quite important. We suggest that you give teachers a short time at the beginning of each new school year to get to know your son or daughter. Then, schedule a meeting with all your child's teachers to discuss your child's strengths and weaknesses. If some particular classroom strategy has worked with your child in the past, let teachers know. You should also be prepared to talk about your child's particular learning style and to plan ways in which you can ensure future communication with school staff. If there are outside professionals working with your son or daughter, inform the school of their existence and encourage communication.

Parents need to establish and maintain good communication channels with school personnel.

In fact, parents need to establish and maintain good communication channels with school personnel. If your child is young and has only one teacher, you can communicate regularly by phone or e-mail. With older children who have several teachers, you may have to develop a formal system with a guidance counselor or have a specific teacher serve as a liaison or coordinator. Do remember that teachers want children to succeed and, in most cases, they have the best intentions when it comes to a child's education. If at all possible, teachers should be viewed as allies, not enemies. When parents and teachers are seen as team players, school staff will try hard to work with a family's goals and expectations. Hopefully, you will have the school's support, but remember that no one will take as much interest in your child as you do. Because you are your child's best advocate, it is very important that you stay on top of your child's academic situation.

77. What kind of teaching styles might be best for my ADHD child?

ADHD children perform best with a structured yet nurturing approach in the classroom. Teachers should be encouraged to make goals and expectations quite explicit. As ADHD children have some specialized needs, your child's teacher should be open to providing and managing individualized programming as well as accepting and understanding the need for accommodations. Any classroom teacher should be skilled in implementing a behavior modification program if it becomes necessary to decrease unwanted behaviors that interfere with your child's learning.

ADHD children perform best with a structured yet nurturing approach in the classroom.

For you as a parent, it is important to work with school administrators to identify the specific teachers who would be the "best fit" for your child. Some teachers, for example, can more easily tolerate the disorganization, impulsivity, and fidgetiness of hyperactive ADHD children. In contrast, some mainstream teachers do not have the skills, experience, or interest in the special education techniques that may be necessary for behavioral or academic intervention with an ADHD student. Be sure your child's specific needs are clearly defined and considered when class placement decisions are made.

78. How do I know whether my child needs specific accommodations or a special education program?

Some children, particularly those with mild to moderate ADHD symptoms, may do quite well in the classroom with only the benefit of medication. Others may need more active accommodations or even special education placement. This is the time when listening to your child and school staff is very important. Parents should carefully peruse their child's grade card and watch for cues at parent–teacher conferences. Try to get to the bottom of teacher comments. Find out how much of the problem is the particular curriculum, a bad teacher–student match, or the direct result of your child's academic performance or poor behavior. If children have accommodations but are still experiencing academic, emotional, or social difficulties in the mainstream classroom that are overwhelming their ability to learn, it may be time to consider a special education classroom where individual needs can be more directly addressed. In a special education setting, the teacher will be responsible for fewer children and will have a greater opportunity to use specialized skills to help students input, understand, integrate, and process information in a better way.

Another crucial point for you to realize is that a child's academic needs may vary over time. Thus, while you may have a good understanding of your child's school-based needs at any given point, it is important that you and school authorities stay open to frequent reevaluation. Be prepared to respond to changing demands, expectations, and needs on all sides—your child's, the school's, and your own.

79. What accommodations should I encourage the school to make for my ADHD child?

Reasonable accommodations are things school personnel can do to make learning and the demonstration of that learning easier for your child. These arrangements include adaptations or adjustments in the way information is presented or expressed in the classroom. School authorities can make changes in what is required to be learned and in how something is taught.

Some school accommodations are commonly made for students with disabilities. These include:

- *Note-taking accommodations*: ADHD students frequently have difficulty with taking notes in an organized and useful fashion. Parents can request that ADHD children use a tape recorder in the classroom so that they can listen a second time to a lecture and refine their classroom notes. Often, they can ask teachers to provide outlines of their lectures to be used as basic skeletal structures for note-taking. Sometimes they can request that school personnel help the student to develop a buddy system whereby two students exchange notes or one student receives a copy of another student's notes. In some cases, particularly in more advanced classes where accurate note-taking is very important, parents can request that someone act as the child's note-taker.
- *Test-taking accommodations*: ADHD students commonly request additional time for completing classroom examinations or standardized testing, such as the SAT. In addition, to minimize distractions, an ADHD student may ask to take an examination in a quiet area of the room or even in a separate room. Students with additional disabilities may request such arrangements as having the test read aloud or employing the services of a scribe.
- *Materials*: ADHD students may ask for an extra set of books to keep at home, thereby avoiding the constant pressure of remembering to bring home all required texts. In addition, if reading a great deal of written material is problematic for ADHD students,

they may request "books on tape" to help to decrease the chance of distraction. Using a laptop computer can also be helpful for ADHD students, particularly when they display visual-organizational or visual-motor difficulties. Other accommodations include using a calculator or dictionary in class.

- *Time*: Time management issues are a common concern for ADHD students. They may need additional time at their locker between classes to sort through their backpacks or get needed materials that may be buried deep at the bottom of their locker. They may also require additional time to get from class to class. Sometimes, designating a specific traveling buddy, who is less apt to be distracted or taken off course on the way to class, can be a good idea. Generally, ADHD students can always benefit from instruction on how to prioritize and manage their time. Have the school delegate a "point person" who, on a daily or weekly basis, can assist an ADHD student in scheduling, managing, and prioritizing assignments and responsibilities, both academic and extra-curricular. Also, because ADHD children take longer to complete tasks, it is helpful to have the teacher modify homework assignments to cut down the written workload.

- *Classroom adjustments*: Because they are so easily distracted, ADHD students may request a seat in the front of class. In some cases, if learning difficulties or behavioral problems dominate, it may be necessary to request an aide. With an additional person in the classroom to serve as a role-model and provide emotional support, ADHD children can learn better techniques for monitoring and controlling their own behavior. Generally, the aide serves as an additional teacher in the classroom, monitoring and intervening when necessary. Other children are often unaware of which student the aide is responsible for.

- *Communication*: Parents and teachers need to work together to help ADHD children. A routine form of communication, such as e-mail or a written log that travels between school and home, can be used to keep parents informed about how their child is performing on a day-to-day basis and about whether they are completing and submitting homework assignments. In that way, parents do not have to wait until the grade card comes home to find out about problems that could have been avoided.

80. What process should I follow to get special education services for my child?

Although the laws vary from state to state, schools usually follow a general format. Most often, a committee on special education (CSE) receives a formal request for an evaluation or for particular remedial services. The request may come from a parent or it may originate with a teacher. School authorities, with parental permission, then conduct a formal assessment. This may consist of questionnaires, standardized tests, classroom observation, or interviews. A family may also choose to finance an evaluation privately outside the school system. This private assessment may substitute for school testing or it may be administered in addition to a child's school system evaluation. Next, parents, teachers, evaluators, and support staff will meet to present findings and make recommendations. At this meeting, participants may come to a consensus about a possible diagnosis or about suggestions for remedial services and accommodations. After such a meeting, the authorities will draw up an individualized education program (IEP) and send it to the parents for their approval and signature.

81. What is an IEP, and why do ADHD students need one?

IEP

An Individualized Educational Program, or IEP, is a written document that is required for every disabled student who is found to meet the federal and state requirements for special education.

The IEP is a written document with several required parts that describe the educational plan for students with a disability.

The acronym **IEP** stands for "individualized education program." The IEP is a written document with several required parts that describe the educational plan for students with a disability. This plan is developed and then reviewed and revised by the school on a regular basis. ADHD children's IEPs include a statement about their present level of educational performance, a list of measurable annual goals, and a description of special education and related services. It may also contain program changes or supports that will be provided to such children. Such IEPs will also include the projected date for the beginning of those services and the anticipated frequency, location, and duration of the services. Finally, it will address how the children's progress toward those annual goals will be measured.

An important function of an IEP is to indicate who will be responsible for determining whether annual goals are met. Be very sure that an IEP is both substantive and clear about your child's needs. It will be only as effective as it is specific. Most important, the IEP is not a finalized legal document until it is signed by a child's parents. In other words, parents have the right to object to what is stated in an IEP and to ask for specific changes.

The Individuals with Disabilities Education Act (IDEA) requires that all disabled students who receive special education services have an IEP written just for them. The IEP helps school personnel to meet ADHD children's special needs and helps you participate in the planning of educational goals. An important purpose of the IEP is to make sure that everyone—the child, the family, and school staff—knows what your child's educational program will be.

Essentially, the IEP is a contract with the school system in that it provides oversight and accountability. It lets you know what must be accomplished and that the school system is responsible for accomplishing the specific designated goals set forth in the document.

82. Who comes to an IEP meeting, and what can I expect will happen there?

You and your child are entitled to at least one IEP meeting per year to formulate and revise the child's IEP. The participants in the meeting are the members of your child's educational team. The members of the team include parents, a selection of teachers (both mainstream and special education staff), school counselors or psychologists, and the school's special education representative who is knowledgeable about services and resources. In addition, school authorities may invite other individuals with special expertise (e.g., speech-language therapists, reading consultants, or occupational therapists). You may also invite others whom you or school personnel think can help with the planning of your child's program. Furthermore, another parent of a special education child can be invited to sit in on the meeting as a resource and support for you. Whenever appropriate, your child will be invited to participate in the meeting.

The format of the meeting may look different, depending on the system established by particular school districts. However, generally the IEP meeting begins with a detailed account of your child's progress over the last year. This includes comments from teachers and specialists and a report of assessments by school personnel or outside consultants. Discussion follows about the child's present needs before deciding about appropriate classification and the designation of proper services for the upcoming year.

83. I have heard that my child may qualify as disabled under Section 504 of the Rehabilitation Act of 1973 or the Americans with Disabilities Act. What are these laws? If my child is not eligible for special education services, can accommodations be granted under these laws?

Section 504 of the Rehabilitation Act of 1973 is another important federal law for people with disabilities. Section 504 is a civil rights law. Its broad purpose is to protect disabled individuals from discrimination due to their disabilities. To be eligible for protections under Section 504, a child must have a physical or mental impairment that substantially limits at least one major life activity. The Americans with Disabilities Act (ADA) is a very similar document. It follows the format of Section 504 but broadens the agencies that must comply with the rights and procedures outlined in Section 504.

To be eligible for protections under Section 504, a child must have a physical or mental impairment that substantially limits at least one major life activity.

It is important to realize that Section 504 and ADA do not guarantee direct special education services like those provided by IDEA. Both Section 504 and the ADA protect disabled children from discrimination. In other words, children served under Section 504 and ADA do not have an IEP and are not necessarily entitled to specifically defined services. However, because many ADHD children do not have other diagnosable learning disabilities, Section 504 is a vehicle through which many ADHD students are served.

The law states that reasonable arrangements must be made for disabled students, but what are reasonable arrangements? Common accommodations that are made under Section 504 or ADA include using assistive technology, removing obstacles to effective communication, and altering rules and policies. That may mean granting children additional time for testing or allowing them to use other testing methods. In addition, in some cases, school personnel may change curriculum, materials, or architecture to meet the needs of a disabled student.

Under Section 504, if parents believe that their child has a disability, whether from ADHD or any other limitation, and the school system has reason to believe that the child needs special education or related services, the school is legally bound to evaluate the child to determine whether he or she is disabled as defined by Section 504.

84. Do I need to consult a legal advocate?

If things are going well between you and your school system, you have no need to consult legal counsel. However, if your relationship has become hostile, talking to an attorney or advocate knowledgeable about your child's legal rights might be a good idea. Nevertheless, it is important to note that the presence of legal counsel at an IEP or other school meeting may have undesirable effects. It could make school officials quite defensive and may actually have a negative impact on your future interactions. In other words, you should weigh carefully whether you're serving your child's best interests by bringing out the "big guns." Legal counsel may, however, provide you with very important information if you are fighting for services that you feel your child deserves.

85. My child has been struggling and unhappy for years in the public school system, even with accommodations. What other alternatives do I have?

Alternatives to public education are available; however, the extent of their availability greatly depends on where you live. They may include parochial schools, private schools, special education schools, and even boarding schools. Before making any decision, it is important to consider the pros and cons of each alternative.

First, cost is a factor. Some options are quite expensive, particularly a special education school, which can charge as much as $30,000 or more a year for your child's education. Your school system may or may not pay these costs. If your school officials feel that they can manage your child's issues within their own system, getting payment from them will be difficult and may involve a legal action. If, however, your system is clearly not equipped to handle your child's issues and has demonstrated this over time, you may be able to convince those in charge to pay for your child's education outside their system. It is very important that you understand that this is not a routine matter. Although you may think that school personnel are as committed to your child's education as you are, paying for private education is most certainly a huge investment on their part. Nevertheless, do know that state reimbursements can decrease the burden to a particular school system.

Second, mainstream private schools may have some of the things that you seek but may lack others. Traditionally, private schools have smaller classes and more individualized attention. However, getting your child access to specialized remedial services (e.g., occupational therapy, social skills groups, remedial reading, or a resource room) may be much harder.

Third, different types of schools have their own advantages and disadvantages. For example, children may be in smaller classes in a private school, but they may also be in a much more competitive situation. Subsequently, dealing with a more challenging curriculum and brighter students may negate the relief they receive from being in a smaller class situation. A special education school may provide crucial help with organizational skills, mathematics, or reading strategies but also may serve many children with disabilities more severe than those of your child. A boarding school may have exactly the right ingredients, but attendance there may mean that your child lives away from home far sooner than a parent may desire.

86. My son is a senior in high school. What preparations must he make in order to get appropriate accommodations and services when he gets to college? How do we find out about which college programs are the best for individuals with ADHD?

It is important to think ahead when it comes to preparing your child for college. First, if you are considering obtaining services, it is crucial that you have an up-to-date assessment of your teenager's capabilities. This may be a recent evaluation by the school or a private assessment that has been administered in the last 2 or 3 years. The document needs to state diagnosis and designate the need for specific services. Colleges and universities offer a range of general services and accommodations as well as ones that are more specific to particular learning issues. Most certainly,

Colleges and universities offer a range of general services and accommodations as well as ones that are more specific to particular learning issues.

accommodations such as extended time and distraction-reduced exam sites should be available. In addition, the assistance of an anonymous note-taker or an editing service for written assignments usually can be arranged. Students can also easily get permission to use a tape recorder or gain access to lecture notes.

Different schools have different arrangements. Some may have an Office of Disability Services, while others may have Learning Centers. These are places where students can access services such as study skills classes, tutors, note-takers and editors. It is also the place where students can find counselors who can provide a variety of supports including helping students formulate and follow-up on an academic plan, assisting with time management issues, providing "coaching" or problem-solving, monitoring for stress and teaching stress-reduction techniques, and referring to other mental health professionals when necessary.

There are colleges that solely serve learning disabled and ADHD students, colleges that have specific special education programs within their broader programming, colleges that offer numerous services and accommodations, and colleges that appear to be less open to serving the needs of an ADHD individual. You must check the school's literature, visit the program, and talk to staff as well as students to gain an accurate picture. Some programs will want a report for an ADHD student included in the application; other programs will discuss options once a student is accepted.

In terms of choosing a particular school, it is important to fully discuss the options with your teenager. Remember to consider your child's academic and psychosocial needs. Subsequently, think about academic demands and services as well as living arrangements, channels for social interaction and opportunities for extracurricular activity. Even though you may set your sights on a particular program with multiple services that seems perfect for your student, if your child does not take advantage of the services, the program may not be a good fit. As adolescents will be on their own and the school is not bound to actively supervise or inform parents of their children's progress, college-bound adolescents must be willing to take responsibility for themselves.

PART FIVE

Psychosocial Issues

How should I talk with my child about an ADHD diagnosis?

My child's ADHD really has brought anger and frustration into our family life. What can I do?

Should I let my ADHD teenager drive, knowing that such adolescents have more automobile accidents?

More . . .

87. How should I talk to my child about an ADHD diagnosis?

The issue of talking to your child about a diagnosis of ADHD is an important consideration. How you go about having a discussion and what you choose to discuss depend greatly on your child's age and personality and on your own parenting style. No matter what, do not keep your child in the dark about this diagnosis. ADHD children need to understand what is physically happening to them, why people react so strongly to their behavior, and what actually is and is not under their control.

ADHD children need to understand what is physically happening to them, why people react so strongly to their behavior, and what actually is and is not under their control.

With younger children, we advise that you let them know that they have a medical condition clearly influencing their behavior. Most likely, they have experienced a lack of success when they tried to control some aspect of their behavior. Young children are relieved to know that they are not entirely responsible for all the disruptions and reactions. Young children may be quite ripe for discussion but just unsure about how to start a dialogue. There are many new children's books that are particularly helpful in explaining the causes and characteristics of ADHD to younger children (discussed in the Appendix). Reading about another elementary school-aged child who's repeatedly told to "pay attention" or "stop disrupting the class" is a good way to open a conversation. These books cover many emotionally laden topics—a teacher's reaction to messy desks, the hurt associated with a rejection by friends, or the need for medication visits to the school nurse—that are important to discuss with an elementary school-aged child. Older children may also gain from reading ADHD books that are written for their age level.

Learning about ADHD is an ongoing process. Whereas younger children learn that some things are not within their control, older children may have to learn more about what they *can* control. Teenagers need to understand not only about how ADHD affects their learning and social interactions, but also how to take hold of the reins and help themselves. Adolescents can learn how to advocate for themselves by openly discussing their learning difficulties with teachers and requesting help or accommodations to meet their individual needs. In addition, adolescence is the prime time for experimentation and rule-breaking behavior. Parents and society set the rules but, in the long run, the adolescents make the decisions. Discussions with older students must focus on helping them to learn to make wise choices and to take responsibility for their behavior. Medication issues are particularly important topics to discuss with your teenager. Stimulant medication is a controlled substance. When students graduate from high school, they most likely will become responsible for their medication. For adolescents to understand how to use and not abuse such drugs is crucial.

Most certainly, parents of college-bound students should set a goal of helping their sons or daughters thoroughly understand their personal symptom profile. These teenagers must develop an awareness of their own individual needs so that they can appropriately advocate for themselves in academic as well as work settings. Topics such as time management, classroom accommodations, the multiple distractions of college life, self-esteem and self-advocacy, appropriate storage of medication in a shared living space, and the dangers of medication abuse should be addressed.

88. Now that my child has diagnosed ADHD, should I let other family members and friends know about it?

Although sharing your child's diagnosis with others has both pros and cons, honesty about the diagnosis is what we recommend. In many ways, the situation is similar to receiving any medical diagnosis. If your child received a diagnosis of asthma, you probably would not immediately pick up the phone to inform all your family and friends. However, if a friend or family member comments about your child's behaviors, you might tell them about the diagnosis. In addition, if family members or friends are taking care of your child for an extended period, you'd provide them with the necessary medical information. Similarly, you should inform people in daily contact with your ADHD child—teachers, caretakers, parents of your child's friends—of the diagnosis so as to be helpful if your child's behavior becomes problematic. In today's world, very little stigma is attached to an ADHD diagnosis. If you approach the topic with a respectful and comfortable attitude, so will the friends, family, and professionals involved with your child.

89. Does having ADHD make it more difficult for my child to make and keep friends?

Some ADHD children have difficulty with social relationships. In some cases, ADHD children who are talkative and have many interests may initially make friends easily. However, the same ADHD children may have difficulty in keeping and developing those friendships. Common complaints from younger children focus around the physical manners of their ADHD friends. ADHD children frequently substitute touch for words which can actually lead to both "rough" touch and too many hugs. Subsequently, other children may become uncomfortable with your child's need for physical contact.

As ADHD children get older, they may pay a bigger price for their failure to abide by the social norms.

As activities become more group-oriented, ADHD children may have more trouble participating. The social skills that are routine to others often do not come naturally for ADHD children. They are notorious for interrupting conversations, not knowing how to take turns in a verbal exchange, inappropriately changing topics, or talking on and on. ADHD children may also not be good listeners. These types of communication difficulties may eventually influence their friendships as peers become increasingly impatient with their lack of social ability. In addition, their immaturity, impulsivity, and need to stay at the center of attention are traits that may cause their peers to reject them. This is not to say that every ADHD child has social difficulties. However, it is a frequently reported aspect of the disorder.

90. What kind of therapeutic support would help me most in dealing with my ADHD adolescent's problems at home, at school, and with peers?

Most certainly, not every child with ADHD requires therapy. As stated in previous discussions, medication treatment may suffice for some children, improving their focus and academic success. Nevertheless, many ADHD children struggle not only academically, but also with peers and family. ADHD children can become quite confused and saddened when they experience social interaction difficulties, peer rejection, or academic failures. They can come to internalize a sense of insecurity that arises out of a feeling that they are "bad." Essentially, repeated negative feedback from parents, teachers, and friends can actively feed that insecurity. Some ADHD children defend against these feelings with a false bravado. Other ADHD children make up for their difficulties by using humor and charisma to maintain their social acceptance. However, frequently their problems of distractibility, impulsiveness, and inattention can lead to more social difficulties as their maturing peers develop different expectations about appropriate behavior.

One consequence of these struggles can be changes in mood and self-esteem. Supportive psychotherapy is a perfect forum for dealing with self-esteem issues. In this type of therapy, ADHD children can comfortably gain more insight and understanding. An essential aspect of the therapy should be a psychoeducational element. Educating a child about the signs, causes, and consequences of ADHD is part of the psychotherapeutic process. As children gain more understanding about their own illness, they will be able to appreciate what areas of behavior are truly changeable and can begin to take more control over their actions.

Educating a child about the signs, causes, and consequences of ADHD is part of the psychotherapeutic process.

Cognitive behavioral therapy is a specific way in which ADHD children can change patterns of perception and behavior that negatively impact their lives. Through cognitive behavioral therapy, they can be helped to discover how their thoughts impact their actions and, subsequently, improve their personal relationships as well as tackle the specific day-to-day issues that interfere with their academic and psychosocial success. Once an issue is identified, the therapist can support the child in his efforts to determine the best method to deal with the problem. Clear-cut goals are established and addressed most frequently in a time-limited fashion. An ADHD individual can work on concerns such as poor self-esteem as well as task persistence and completion, disorganization, time management, and follow-through. It is also the setting in which to focus on specific behaviors that may disrupt conversation such as excessive talking, interrupting, and rambling.

Professionally led social skills group meetings are also helpful places for ADHD children to learn how to deal more effectively with the tricky rules of peer relationships. At such gatherings, naturally occurring interactions can be wonderful opportunities to target behaviors and teach appropriate social skills.

91. My child's ADHD really has brought anger and frustration into our family life. What can I do?

For ADHD children, an increasing problem can arise when home, a traditional source of safety and nurture, becomes another area of stress owing to constant conflict with siblings or parents. ADHD children often do not fit into a normative mode of the well-behaved, competent child. They are often quite sensitive about acceptance in all situations and take even minimal criticism as a rebuff. Because ADHD children can demand so much attention, other family members can begin to feel that the entire family revolves around the ADHD child. Siblings can find it particularly tough when they have similar needs but receive less family focus.

Family roles can become rigid and fixed, and changing them can be difficult. For example, a very common role for an ADHD child is to become the "difficult" child in the family. The family puts a great deal of energy and focus into helping such a child fit more appropriately into their family system. Other children can become quite resentful of the attention given to their affected sibling.

Because ADHD children can demand so much attention, other family members can begin to feel that the entire family revolves around the ADHD child.

Subsequently, the family becomes another place in which an ADHD child's negative behavior becomes reinforced because of all the reaction it produces. Even the best-intentioned family may experience difficulty in incorporating the ADHD child into their family system. As a result, instead of feeling safe and comfortable at home, ADHD children may feel isolated and alone within their own family.

Working with a family therapist can be quite helpful. In other therapeutic situations, the ADHD child is deemed the "designated patient." In family therapy, the rules are different. By changing the therapeutic focus to help all family members to express their individual needs, improve their communication skills, set appropriate expectations, and become more functional as a family unit, the entire family becomes the patient.

No doubt having an ADHD child can put a great deal of pressure on a marriage. These often "high-maintenance" children place stress on couples to be even more unified in their parenting approach and decision-making process. A family therapist may work specifically with the parents to help them communicate more effectively with each other, to assess situations, to set appropriate rules and boundaries, to manage family conflicts, and to make decisions.

Another option for parents is a parent support group. There are many of these "self-help" groups throughout the country (see the Appendix). They provide a wonderful opportunity for parents to meet with others who share similar questions and concerns about their ADHD child. Sharing stories can greatly lessen the isolation and stress. At the same time, there are many occasions to learn from the experiences of others.

92. What is the best way to discipline my ADHD child for behavior problems? Should I set more limits?

Most professionals will emphasize that it is very important for parents of ADHD children to establish clear rules and consequences for breaking those rules. A behavior management program will most likely be a great benefit to children who break the rules and exhibit inappropriate behaviors. This type of program is based on a reward system in which parents highlight and reinforce specific behaviors to help such children make desired behaviors more automatic. Under this system, parents either ignore or negatively reward other, more problematic behaviors. Frequently, such children earn points, working toward a designated goal or reward. The objective of such a system is to establish a pattern of behavior in the home that can then be extended to the outside world.

Some pointers for any program include such things as making sure that your ADHD child is paying attention when you discuss the rules. Although this is true in general, it's particularly important when you're going out in public places. Define expectations before you go out by making a plan that you're sure your child understands. Also, in developing any behavior management plan, be sure that the negative consequences are as clearly defined as the rewards.

When you show approval to ADHD children, be sure to be direct, using both verbalizations and gestures so that they clearly understand the message. In addition, be sure that inherent in your program is a structure that not only weeds out unwanted behavior but teaches new positive behavior. In other words, the fact that children learn not to interrupt someone when they want to enter a conversation does not necessarily mean that they know the right way to enter a group discussion. You need to specifically teach ADHD children certain behaviors that many children learn as a natural part of their developmental process. The important lesson here is not to expect what can not be delivered.

93. Must I see a therapist to begin a behavior management program at home, or can I do it myself?

Online parent sites can be very helpful in giving you some ideas about how to start your own behavioral program. There are also many books on the subject (see the Appendix). However, if you feel that the world of "behavior management" is too complicated and overwhelming, you can find a professional to work with you. In addition, parents often find it difficult to maintain objectivity, particularly when they are in the midst of a crisis and having a hard time managing their child. Parents can easily find themselves in a situation in which they are responding only to the unwanted behavior, forming a destructive negative feedback loop between parent and child. However, that is just the time when parents may need a behavioral plan. At those times, outside guidance of some sort may actually be quite useful in helping parents get started.

94. My ADHD child is a teenager. Is behavior management different with adolescents?

Professionals suggest that ADHD teenagers should take a more active role in designing a plan for resolving conflicts. In other words, you and your child need to mutually define problems (e.g., provide both sides of the curfew dilemma). Then, the task becomes one in which you and your child work together to generate possible solutions and evaluate the alternatives. Finally, you can come to an understanding about a mutually agreed-upon solution. Ideally, this gives teenagers more control in the process. In that way, they also learn a pattern of behavior that they can carry out for themselves.

95. My teenager always appears unmotivated and apathetic. Is this common in ADHD?

Many ADHD teenagers have had the experience of working quite hard to reap very few rewards within the academic system. They become frustrated and exhausted in their efforts to keep up with the successes of their peers. Apathy is one route that routinely unsuccessful children may choose to take. Instead of trying to meet external or internal demands, they grow increasingly apathetic and unmotivated. Essentially, if they do not attempt to succeed, they can not blame failure on a lack of ability. "I didn't try, so of course I failed" is their face-saving strategy.

However, apathy can also be a sign of comorbid depression. If ADHD children routinely meet failure in school, it is crucial that steps be taken to meet with school staff, obtain specific remedial help, make accommodations, or transfer to a more appropriate academic setting. If these types of interventions do not succeed, a psychiatric evaluation may be necessary.

96. Many teenagers experiment with drugs and alcohol. Is my ADHD adolescent more at risk for this kind of problematic behavior?

Because many ADHD children are impulsive and need attention, they definitely are more prone to engage in risky behavior. Sometimes, on the social fringe, using drugs is a way in which they can seem to join the crowd. Often, the immediate rewards of the activity move to the forefront, and children do not stop to think about the consequences of their actions. In addition, some professionals feel that ADHD children are at great risk of abusing drugs, particularly marijuana.

This is an area in which parents need to try to keep up communication with their adolescents. Discussions about peer pressure are very important. Teenagers can also benefit from practicing how to say "no" to their friends. If, however, you feel that your child may be regularly using or abusing drugs, you should talk to a professional and develop a drug screening program that you can use at home. This may mean that you have to intermittently and unexpectedly ask for a urine sample from your child. This approach can precipitate a conflict between you and your child, which is why professional support is necessary.

97. Should I let my ADHD teenager drive, knowing that such adolescents have more automobile accidents?

It is true that ADHD teenagers have both a higher rate of ticketing and a higher rate of accidents as compared to non-ADHD adolescents. The literature suggests that most likely poor "self-control" is at the root of ADHD teenagers' predisposition toward poor driving. As in other areas of functioning, ADHD teens tend to act before thinking when they are driving. This impulsivity increases their risk of motor vehicle crashes and violations. However, ADHD teenagers *will* become drivers. The important issue is how parents can help their teens to develop safe driving habits. In other words, how can parents decrease the chances that their ADHD child will be involved in an automobile accident?

Some suggestions can help to make driving safe:

- *Instruction:* If possible, have your teenager receive professional instruction. A wide variety of driver's education programs are connected to the schools and private driving instructors are available. Taking parents out of the primary instructor role has benefits. First, objective driving programs require your child to cover all the basics in a highly organized, structured fashion. Second, you can avoid a lot of the heated battles between parent and child that can arise in new driving situations. Third, an objective person is evaluating and critiquing your child's driving skills. However, whether you're the primary or secondary driving instructor, remember that patience is essential. Schedule regular, well-planned driving lessons. As with homework, think "short and frequent" so that your teenager is able to accumulate plenty of supervised driving time.
- *Driving rules:* Be very clear with your teenager about the driving rules. Strictly impose "no-drinking-and-driving" rules. Prohibit late-night driving until your teenager is very experienced. Consider how many other teenagers you will allow in your car with your teenage driver. Remember, the presence of other adolescents in the car will be more likely to distract your teenager.
- *Consequences:* Immediate consequences for poor driving performance or broken driving rules are crucial. Parents should remind ADHD teenagers that behind the wheel, they are responsible not only for themselves but also for passengers, other drivers, and pedestrians. Your teenager will better understand the importance of safe driving if you firmly and clearly stand by your rules for responsible driving behavior.

- *Medication:* Studies suggest that teenagers drive more safely when they've taken their medication. Most certainly, medication can be very helpful when adolescents are first learning to drive. At that point, important details and distractions can be particularly overwhelming. However, as teenagers drive for longer periods and at later hours, the medication issue becomes more complicated. Nevertheless, keep driving safety in mind when you and your teen decide the details of a medication regimen.

No doubt all parents struggle with issues surrounding safe teenage driving; however, the problem can be even more difficult for parents of ADHD teens. Not only are parents confronted with increased safety risks, but they sometimes have a stubborn child who has a hard time accepting the rules.

98. I know that I need to let my teenager be responsible for himself as he moves on to college and, eventually, independent living. But what if I sense that he is beginning to do poorly? At what point should I intervene?

Many ADHD students will find great success at college. Nevertheless, others may find themselves walking a rocky road. Some ADHD students want a fresh start when they head off to college. They have felt burdened by being identified as "disabled" in high school and now just want to be like everyone else. Therefore, they may refuse services and/or medication. Other students go off with the best intentions to use available resources and/or manage their time appropriately, yet are unable to actively assert themselves within the peer environment or successfully advocate for their own needs. Others may just become overwhelmed by the amount of work, the multiple distractions, and the lack of parental guidance. Because some of these students have been "micro-managed" by parents during their high school years, it may be quite difficult for them to now operate more independently. Subsequently, some of these students may find themselves falling behind academically.

Fortunately or unfortunately, you cannot accompany your college student on his journey down this road. This fact is reinforced by the college's privacy rules which make it difficult for parents to talk to counselors or gain access to information about students' progress. Therefore, keeping an open channel of communication with your college student is the best approach. It is important to remember that even students without learning issues often take more than 4 years to complete college. Your ADHD teenager may choose to enroll for a reduced course-load, take off for a semester or a year, or live at home while attending school as a full-time or part-time student. In other words, ADHD students may have to find their own educational pace and rhythm. Some of these students may stumble along the way; however, by pulling themselves up and finding a means to move forward, they only increase their opportunity for success.

For that group of ADHD individuals whose symptoms persist into adulthood, an important thing to realize is that ADHD may continue to affect their social and vocational interactions even though their days of academic performance have passed. Although they may have focused in their youth on school success, problems with inattention, impulsivity, irritability, and disorganization can continue. That's partly why psychotherapeutic intervention and medication as treatment are so crucial for ADHD individuals. Young adults who are armed with increased awareness of their disorder and a true

Young adults who are armed with increased awareness of their disorder and a true appreciation of their own limitations have a better chance of success in today's world.

appreciation of their own limitations have a better chance of success in today's world. Parents must learn to speak honestly when things appear to go badly; however, their capacity to intervene becomes significantly less as ADHD children become adults.

99. What is the likelihood that a biological marker will be developed?

The development of tests to diagnose ADHD objectively is definitely on the horizon. Discovering the gene or genes responsible for ADHD will permit more exact diagnosis. Imaging studies that document neurotransmitter function, for example, map and measure dopamine levels that may eventually provide objective evidence of ADHD. Imaging studies that show which areas of brain are active during particular activities—especially those that are problematic for children with ADHD—may turn out to be a useful way to diagnose ADHD. Certain structures like the frontal lobes, striatum, and the cerebellum appear to be smaller in individuals with ADHD. In the future, we may be able to easily measure the size of these structures on routine MRI and use this information as a clinical tool for diagnosis.

100. Where can I get more information about ADHD?

The Appendix that follows provides a number of resources for parents of ADHD children, adults with ADHD, and others interested in this topic. It includes books, agency contact information, and Internet sites. When using the Internet, remember that not all information you find there is accurate, scientific, or up-to-date. You need to be astute about your use of Internet information. If in doubt, look to a personal contact for professional resources.

Resources for Parents

Parent Groups

Children and Adults with Attention Deficit Disorders (CHADD)
8181 Professional Place, Suite 201
Landover, MD 20785
Phone: 1-800-233-4050
Web: www.chadd.org
CHADD provides family support and advocacy, public and professional educa-
tion, and encouragement of scientific research on ADHD. Information about
local CHADD chapters is available on the Web. Contains a good newsletter.

Learning Disabilities Association of America (LDA)
4156 Library Road
Pittsburgh, PA 15234
Phone: 412-341-1515 or 412-341-8077
Fax: 412-344-0224
E-mail: info@LDAAmerica.org
Web: www.ldanatl.org

National Attention Deficit Disorder Association (National ADDA)
1788 Second Street, Suite 200
Highland Park, IL 60035
Phone: 847-432-ADDA
Web: www.add.org
National ADDA places particular emphasis on young adults with ADD, focusing
on issues of work, career, college, and other forms of higher education in addition
to legal matters and relationships. Information on local ADDA chapters is available on the Web. Contains a good newsletter.

National Center for Learning Disabilities
381 Park Avenue South, Suite 1401
New York, NY 10016
Phone: 212-545-7510 or 1-888-575-7373
Fax: 212-545-9665
Web: www.ncld.org

General ADHD Websites: Online Communities and Resources

http://www.addhelpline.org/parentsmenu.htm
This online site has a chat room, newsletter, motivational and parenting tips,
and columns by coaches who specialize in ADHD. Resources also include a
weekly online support meeting.

http://www.ldonline.org/adhdbasics
This online site contains helpful, easy-to-read information about ADHD, and it
provides some good tips for people struggling with ADHD of all ages.

*http://www.aboutourkids.org/families/disorders_treatments/az_disorder_guide/
attentiondeficithyperactivity_disorder*
NYU Child Study Center Website that contains a variety of helpful information
about ADHD along with some videos. The website also provides parents with
a number of more recent articles about ADHD, in addition to treatment and
research options at NYU CSC.

www.addvance.com
A website created by Patricia Quinn, MD and Kathleen Nadeau, PhD. Both are
internationally recognized as ADD specialists and have written a number of
books on the disorder. There is a special section of the Website geared toward
women and girls that may be of interest.

http://www.nimh.nih.gov/health/publications/attention-deficit-hyperactivity-disorder/complete-index.shtml
NIMH's Website on ADHD outlines a great deal of basic information about causes and treatment of ADHD and provides readers with a list of recent scholarly articles concerning the disorder.

Drug Company–Sponsored Websites

www.adhdsupportcompany.com
Shire Pharmaceuticals ADHD Website. An interesting, easily accessible Website with a wealth of information from personal testimonials about living with ADHD to suggestions for helping your child manage his ADHD symptoms.

www.strattera.com
Strattera's Website offers help for both children and adults with ADHD.

Books and Articles about Homework

The Homework Organizer: Assignment Notebook and Guide. G.E. Mengel. South Hadley, MA: Get Organized, 1993. Phone: 800-944-6886.

Homework Partners: Study Buddies: Parent Tutoring Tactics. J. Bowen, D. Olympia, W. Jenson. Longmont, CO: Sopris West, 1996–1998. Phone: 303-651-2829.

Homework Success for Children with ADHD: A Family-School Intervention Program. Thomas Power, PhD, J. Karustis, D. Habboushe. New York: Guilford Press, 2001.

Seven Tips for Homework Success. A Detailed Guide to Get You through Homework. S.S. Zentall, S. Goldstein. Plantation, FL: Specialty Press, 1999.

Books for Children with ADHD

All Dogs Have ADHD. K. Hoopmann. London, UK: Jessica Kingsley Publishers, 2009.

Cory Stories: A Kid's Book about Living With ADHD. J. Kraus. Washington, DC: Magination Press, 2004.

Help4ADD. K. Nadeau. Bethesda, MD: Advantage Books, 1998.
This book was written for teenagers with ADHD. It is designed like a Website. It has short, easy-to-read, information-packed sections about how to get your

Appendix

life together—for yourself, not for your parents or teachers. It has tips about studying, ways in which your high school can help you succeed, and tips about getting along better at home, dating, and exercise.

I Would If I Could. M. Gordon. DeWitt, NY: Gordon Systems, 1992.
Written from a child's perspective, this book offers both humor and sensitivity.

Learning to Slow Down and Pay Attention: A Book for Kids about ADHD.
  K. Nadeau, D. Dixon. Washington, DC: Magination Press, 1997.
This book is fast-paced and funny. It discusses the symptoms of ADHD and
  some possible solutions. It is aimed at younger elementary school-age children
  and some older children who have short attention spans.

Otto Learns about His Medicine. M. Galvin. Washington, DC: American
  Psychological Association, 1995.
This illustrated book uses the metaphor of a car engine's speed and the mechanics'
  work on it to explain ADHD to elementary school children.

Putting on the Brakes. P. Quinn, J Stern. Washington, DC: American Psychological Association, 1991.
This book explains the definition of ADHD and gives information about how
  to improve problem areas, such as organization. Children will be able to read
  this and know what ADHD is and what they can do to help themselves. It
  has tips about making friends, getting organized, and even about medication.
  This book is for the older elementary school and middle school children ages
  8 to 13 years. Parents and children can use this book together.

Some Kids Just Can't Sit Still! S. Goldstein. Plantation, FL: Specialty
  Press/A.D.D. Warehouse, 2009.

Sparky's Excellent Misadventures: My A.D.D. Journal. P. Carpente.
  Washington, DC: Magination Press, 1999.

The Survival Guide for Kids with ADD or ADHD. J. Taylor. Minneapolis,
  MN: Free Spirit Publishing, Inc., 2006.

Books for College Students
**ADD and the College Student: A Guide for High School and College
  Students with Attention Deficit Disorder**. P. Quinn. Washington, DC:
  Magination Press, 2001.

Coaching College Students with AD/HD. P. Quinn, N. Ratey, T. Maitland. Washington, DC: Advantage Books, 2000.
An informative text for parents of college students with ADHD, and for the students themselves, on surviving in the university environment with ADHD.

College Confidence with ADD, M. Sandler. Naperville, IL: Sourcebooks, Inc., 2008.
From application through graduation, this manual provides the ADD student with important information on handling academic as well as social challenges of college life.

Survival Guide for College Students with ADHD or LD, Second Edition. K. Nadeau. Washington, DC: Magination Press, 2006.
The book is written for young adults who have ADHD or learning disabilities and are heading off to college. This book has lots of tips for success in the college setting, which can often prove daunting to those with ADHD.

Unlocking Potential: College and Other Choices for People with LD and AD/HD. Edited by J. Taymans, L. West, M. Sullivan, B. Scheiber. Bethesda, MD: Woodbine House, 2000.

General Books about ADHD for Parents

The ADHD Parenting Handbook: Practical Advice for Parents from Parents. C. Alexander-Roberts. Dallas, TX: Taylor Publishing Company, 1994.

The Attention Zone: A Parent's Guide to Attention Deficit/Hyperactivity. M. Cohen. Philadelphia, PA: Taylor & Francis, 1998.

Born to Be Wild: Attention Deficit Hyperactivity Disorder, Alcoholism, and Addiction. W. Beyer, R.D. Hunt. Midlothian, VA: Judy Wood, 1999.
A guide for parents about ADHD and the potential relationship between ADHD and substance abuse and addictions. Instructions about educational, medical, and family management are included.

Driven to Distraction: Recognizing and Coping with Attention Deficit Disorder from Childhood through Adulthood. E.M. Hallowell, J.J. Ratey. New York: Touchstone, 1994.
Through vivid stories of the experiences of their patients (both adults and children), the authors show the varied forms ADD takes—from the hyperactive search for high stimulation to the floating inattention of daydreaming—and the transforming impact of precise diagnosis and treatment. The authors

explain when and how medication can be extraordinarily helpful and, because both have ADD, their advice on effective behavior-modification techniques for overcoming the syndrome is enriched by their own experience.

From Chaos to Calm: Effective Parenting of Challenging Children with ADHD and Other Behavioral Problems. J.E. Heininger, S.K. Weiss. New York: Perigee Books, 2001.
This book offers practical solutions for parents who are raising a challenging child.

Parenting Children with ADHD: 10 Lessons That Medicine Cannot Teach. V. Monastra. Washington, DC: American Psychological Association, 2004.

Straight Talk about Psychiatric Medications for Kids. T.E. Wilens. New York: Guilford Press 2002.
With numerous real-life examples, answers to frequently asked questions, and helpful tables and charts, Harvard University researcher and practitioner Timothy E. Wilens explains which medications may be prescribed for children, and why; examines effects on children's health, emotions, and school performance; separates facts from myths; and helps parents become active, informed managers of their child's care.

Taking Charge of ADHD. R. Barkley. New York: Guilford Press, 2000.
This is a great book for tips about bringing up the child with ADHD. It provides readers with scientific, historical, and practical information about the disorder and advice and resources for dealing with it.

Your Defiant Child: Eight Steps to Better Behavior. R.A. Barkley, C.M. Benton. New York: Guilford Press, 1999.
This book helps concerned parents understand what causes child defiance, when it becomes a problem, and how it can be resolved. Its clear eight-step program stresses consistency and cooperation, promoting changes through a system of praise, rewards, and mild punishment. Readers benefit from concrete guidelines for establishing clear patterns of discipline, communicating with children on a level they can understand, and reducing family stress overall.

Newsletters

Brakes: The Interactive Newsletter for Kids with ADD. J. Stern, P. Stern, eds. Washington, DC: American Psychological Association Press.
Phone: 202-336-5500.
A newsletter dedicated specifically to children and early adolescents with ADHD. Each issue is filled with information about entertaining activities for children.

CHADD Newsletter. Landover, MD: CHADD National Headquarters. Phone: 301-306-7070; Fax: 301-306-7090.

A newsletter for parents of children with ADHD and adults with ADHD who are members of CHADD.

Videotapes for Parents and Kids

ADD in the 21st Century

A video series on ADD featuring Edward Hallowell, MD and hosted by Dr. Peter Salgo, Emmy Award-Winning Health and Medical Correspondent. This series contains "Kids & ADD" (55 min) and "ADD Goes to School" (45 min). 2 Video Set, $75.00.

ADD—From A To Z. Understanding the Diagnosis and Treatment of Attention Deficit Disorder in Children and Adults.

Can be purchased on www.drhallowell.com/store/index.html. Video, lecture format, $39.95.

ADHD—What Do We Know? ADHD—What Can We Do? ADHD in the Classroom. ADHD in Adults. R.A. Barkley. New York: Guilford Press. Phone: 800-365-7006.

Four award-winning videotapes on ADHD spanning a variety of topics and using children and adults with ADHD who tell their own stories about living with ADHD.

Assessing ADHD in the Schools and Classroom Interventions for ADHD.

G. DuPaul, G. Stoner. New York: Guilford Press. Phone: 800-365-7006.

Excellent videos for school professionals on the specific methods recommended for school-based assessment of children with ADHD and specific methods on classroom management for such children.

It's Just an Attention Disorder, Why Won't My Child Pay Attention? Educating Inattentive Children. S. Goldstein, M. Goldstein. Salt Lake City, UT: Neurology, Learning and Behavior Center. Phone: 801-532-1484.

The first videotape is an excellent introduction to ADHD, intended for older children and teens with ADHD. It has a fast-paced format and uses comments from teens with ADHD about coping with their disorder. The second and third videotapes are intended for viewing by parents and teachers, respectively, and provide a fine overview of the disorder and its management at home and school.

Jumping Johnny, Get Back to Work! M. Gordon. DeWitt, NY: Gordon
Systems, Inc., Phone: 315-446-4849.
An excellent animated video for children with ADHD that discusses the
disorder and its treatment from a child's perspective.

Understanding the Defiant Child. Managing the Defiant Child. R.A. Barkley.
New York: Guilford Press. Phone: 800-365-7006.
These two videos complement the parent-training program described in *Your
Defiant Child* (see General Books About ADHD for Parents). They provide
a clear concise understanding of the factors that contribute to defiance in
children, and specific methods parents can employ to reduce it and improve
parent-child relationships.

Disability and Special Education Resources

The Council for Exceptional Children (CEC)
Phone: 888-CEC-SPED
Fax: 703-264-9494
Web: www.cec.sped.org
The Council for Exceptional Children (CEC) is the largest international professional organization dedicated to improving educational outcomes for individuals with exceptionalities, students with disabilities, or gifted students. CEC
advocates for appropriate governmental policies, sets professional standards,
provides continual professional development, advocates for underserved individuals with exceptionalities, and helps professionals to obtain conditions and
resources necessary for effective professional practice.

Federal Resource Center for Special Education (FRC)
Academy for Educational Development
1825 Connecticut Avenue, NW
Washington, DC 20009
Phone: 202-884-8215
Web: www.dssc.org/frc/index.htm
The FRC is a five-year contract between the Academy for Educational Devel-
opment (AED), its partner, the National Association of State Directors of
Special Education (NASDSE), and the U.S. Department of Education,
Office of Special Education Programs (OSEP). The FRC supports a nation-
wide technical assistance network to respond to the needs of students with
disabilities, especially students from underrepresented populations. The six
regional resource centers (RRCs) are specifically funded to assist state education agencies in the systemic improvement of education programs, practices,
and policies that affect children and youth with disabilities.

The National Information Center for Children and Youth with Disabilities (NICHCY)
PO Box 1492
Washington, DC 20013
Phone: 800-695-0285
Web: www.nichcy.org
NICHCY is the national information and referral center that provides information about disabilities and disability-related issues for families, educators, and other professionals focusing on children and youth, from birth to age 22 years. NICHCY publishes free, fact-filled newsletters, arranges workshops, and advises parents about the laws entitling children with disabilities to special education and other services. State resource sheets—also available online—will help you to locate organizations and agencies within your state that address disability-related issues.

Glossary

Addiction: A pattern of drug abuse characterized by compulsive use of a drug and an excessive focus on getting a supply of a drug to the extent that is psychologically and/or physically habit-forming.

Agonist: A medication that has the same action as the natural neurotransmitter.

Antidepressants: Medications used to treat depression (e.g., Prozac, Wellbutrin, or Effexor).

Basal ganglia: Also referred to as the striatum, the basal ganglia is a group of interconnected nuclei that lie deep within the brain that include the caudate, putamen, globus pallidus, and thalamus. Each of the nuclei (and its connections to other brain structures) appears to be more or less involved in various disorders, such as ADHD, tics, Parkinson's disease, and chorea.

Biofeedback: A method of treatment that uses monitors to feedback to individuals physiological information, such as blood pressure or heart rate, of which they are normally unaware. Through this process, individuals can learn to adjust their thinking in an effort to better control their bodies.

Bipolar disorder: Mood disorder characterized by alternating depressive and manic symptoms.

Caudate: Nucleus within the basal ganglia that appears to be most involved in ADHD. It is rich in dopamine and about 5% smaller in children with ADHD.

Cerebellum: A brain structure in the hindbrain that is primarily involved in balance and coordination. Its role in cognitive and behavior disorders, including ADHD, has been recently discovered.

Clinical trial: A carefully monitored study of a drug or a treatment using a drug that involves a large group of people with the goal of testing that drug's effectiveness.

Cognitive: Pertaining to cognition, the process of knowing and, more precisely, the process of being aware, thinking, learning, and judging.

Comorbidity: Presence of two or more disorders in the same individual.

Conduct disorder: A disorder in which there is an active transgression of societal rules.

Corpus callosum: A structure that lies between the left and right hemisphere and is required for passing information between them. A role for the corpus callosum in ADHD has been recently hypothesized because it tends to be smaller than normal in children with ADHD by about 5%.

Cross-over study: A study in which the subject takes one treatment for part of the study period and another treatment for the other part of the study period. Usually one treatment is the drug being tested and the other treatment is a placebo.

Dependence: The physical need for the repeatedly used and abused drug to the point where withdrawal symptoms will appear if the drug is stopped.

Dopamine transporter (DAT): An enzyme that transports dopamine back into the presynaptic neuron, lowering the level of dopamine in the synaptic space.

Double-blind: A study in which neither the subject nor the investigator know whether the subject is getting the drug or the placebo.

Dyslexia: A specific learning disability marked by impairment in the ability to recognize, read, and process written words.

Electroencephalogram (EEG): A test that measures brain electrical activity.

Enzyme: A protein that controls a chemical reaction in a living organism.

Executive functions: A set of complex behaviors that are necessary for a person to attain goals and adapt to changing environmental demands. They include such brain functions as planning, organizing, initiating, sustaining, shifting, and inhibiting behaviors.

Frontal lobe: The area of the brain that controls executive functions.

Frontostriatal circuit: The connections between the frontal lobes of the brain and the basal ganglia that is located deeper within the brain.

Functional magnetic resonance imaging (fMRI): MRI of the brain done while an activity is being performed that is formatted in a way to show where that activity is happening. For example, an fMRI done during an executive function task will show maximal activity in the frontal lobe.

Gene pool: Genes for different disorders that are more or less common in particular populations.

Gene therapy: A treatment in which an abnormal version of a gene is replaced by a normal version of the gene.

Generic medications: Contain the same ingredients as name brands, but the amount of the ingredient is not as precisely scrutinized. The difference from pill to pill remains minimal.

Generics may also be packaged using different dyes and preservatives. In many instances generics are just as good as the name brand and cost a lot less.

Genetic proclivity: Likelihood that a disorder is passed from one generation to another by a gene or genes.

Half-life: A measure of the duration of a drug's action, how long it takes before one-half the dose is gone. Drugs with long half-lives can be given infrequently, whereas drugs with short half-lives need to be given frequently.

Heritability rate: Reflects the percentage of the cause of ADHD that is attributable to genetic as opposed to environmental factors. A heritability rate of 0.6 means that 60% of the cause of ADHD in an individual is genetic.

Hyperkinetic: The British term for hyperactivity.

IEP: An Individualized Educational Program, or IEP, is a written document that is required for every disabled student who is found to meet the federal and state requirements for special education.

Magnetic resonance imaging (MRI): A technique that creates three-dimensional images of brain structures using strong magnetic fields.

Metabolize: What the body does in reaction to a medication. Some people metabolize relatively slowly or relatively quickly when compared to others. This means that people can require different doses of the same medication to get similar effects.

Motor control: Can describe fine motor control that is needed in handwriting or the gross motor control that is needed to coordinate motor activities such as walking and running. Motor control can also refer to the degree to which a child with ADHD can control his fidgetiness.

MTA study: National Institute of Health-sponsored Multimodal Treatment Study of Children with ADHD. Almost 600 combined-type ADHD children aged 7 to 9 years old were divided into four groups. For just over 1 year, one group received medication monitored by the study researchers, a second group received intensive behavioral therapy, a third group received medication monitored by the study researchers as well as behavioral therapy, and the fourth was given whatever treatment was used in their community, which may or may not have included medication. This group of children has now been followed, some on and some off stimulants for about 3 years, and the outcome has been continually reevaluated.

Neurological: Refers to functions controlled by the brain.

Neurons: Brain cells that can both send and receive information from other brain cells.

Neuropsychological assessment: Series of measures used to examine the behavioral expression of brain function.

Neurotransmitters: Chemical messengers that allow neurons to communicate with one another by transferring information from one brain cell to another. Dopamine, norepinephrine, and serotonin are neurotransmitters implicated in ADHD.

Obsessive-compulsive disorder: A disorder in which individuals experience obsessions and/or compulsions.

Occipital lobe: Area of the brain that controls vision.

Oppositional defiant disorder: Disorder characterized by negative, hostile, and defiant behavior that causes significant damage in social, academic, or occupational interactions.

Parietal lobe: Area of the brain that controls sensory motor skills and also serves to integrate multiple sensory capacities such as tactile (touch) and auditory (hearing) functions.

Placebo: "Sugar pills" used in a clinical trial to identify whether the subject is responding just to the act of taking a pill or to the medication being tested.

Postsynaptic neuron: Receives the message carried by the neurotransmitter.

Presynaptic neuron: Sends the message by releasing a neurotransmitter.

Psychosocial: Involving the psychological and social aspects of mental health.

Rebound: Undesirable irritability, moodiness, fatigue, or hyperactivity as stimulant medicine wears off. It can usually be mitigated by medication adjustment.

Receptor sites: Places on neurons that bind neurotransmitters or where medications act. Some medications can increase or decrease the number or sensitivity of receptors.

Selective serotonin reuptake inhibitors (SSRIs): Medications that work by inhibiting the serotonin transporter. Therefore serotonin, which would ordinarily be shuttled into the neuron, remains in the synapse for a longer period of time, until it diffuses away or is destroyed by an enzyme.

Stimulants: Medications like Ritalin and Adderall that are used to treat ADHD and work primarily by changing dopamine levels.

Striatum: Part of the basal ganglia, which consists of several interconnected regions/nuclei deep within the brain, specifically the caudate and putamen.

Subclinical: A form of a disease with very mild symptoms, often barely noticeable. In inherited disorders, family members who must be affected based on the genetic pattern of the disease, but who do not appear too obviously affected, are described as having subclinical symptoms.

Substance abuse: Self-administration of any drug in a culturally disapproved manner that has adverse consequences.

Synapse: Specialized site between two neurons (brain cells) where neurotransmitters can pass from one cell to the next.

Temporal lobe: Area of the brain that controls memory and language skills.

Tics: Involuntary muscle movements or twitches like blinking, eye rolling, or shoulder shrugging.

Tourette's syndrome: A disorder characterized by motor and vocal tics. To be diagnosed with Tourette's, tics must be present for at least 1 year.

Vocal tics: Involuntary sounds such as throat clearing, sniffing, or words.

Withdrawal: The psychological and/or physical reaction to abruptly stopping a dependence-producing drug.

Glossary

INDEX

A

abuse
    college and stimulant, 92–94
    of stimulants, 78–79
    substance, 24–25
academic accommodations. *See* school accommodations
academic performance, anxiety over, 40–41
ADA. *See* Americans with Disabilities Act
Adderall, 50, 62–63
    dosage of, 57
    Ritalin compared to, 58
Adderall XR, 61, 62
addiction
    dopamine and, 79
    stimulants and, 75–81
ADHD. *See* attention deficit hyperactivity disorder
adolescents
    advocating for themselves, 129
    alcohol/drugs and, 137–138
    apathy and, 137
    behavioral management and, 136–137
    substance abuse and, 24–25
adults, 2–3, 141–142
age
    ADHD occurrence and, 6, 8
    attention expectation by, 46–47
    diagnosis and, 4, 6, 8, 22, 36–37
    symptoms changing with, 22–23
agoraphobia, 40
alcohol
    adolescents and, 137–138
    stimulants and, 85
Americans with Disabilities Act (ADA), 120–121
amphetamine, 50
anemia, iron-deficiency, 21
antidepressants, 50
    tricyclic, 63
anti-tic medications, 50
anxiety disorders, 40–41
apathy, and adolescents, 137
appetite suppression, stimulants and, 66

athletics, 110–111
atomoxetine (Strattera), 50
attention deficit hyperactivity disorder (ADHD)
    age and occurrence of, 6, 8
    attention problems compared to, 25–26
    in birth, 18
    brain damage and, 13–14
    causes of, 2, 16
    celebrities with, 14
    children outgrowing, 8
    children with, 2
    diagnosis of, 3, 28–47
    dopamine transmission in, 11–12
    educational benefits with, 35–36
    environmental factors impacting, 20
    frequency of, 2–5
    gender affecting, 26–27
    genes involved in, 12–13, 16–17
    heritability rate and, 16–17
    neurological problems causing, 17
    OCD diagnosis with, 41–42
    psychosocial problems causing, 17
    risk factors of, 16–22
    subtypes of, 5–6
    symptoms of, 7, 22–28
    television and, 18–19
    Tourette's syndrome and, 38
    what is, 2
attention problems, ADHD compared to, 25–26
autistic spectrum disorder, 45–46

B

basketball, 110–111
behavior, isolated, 23–24
behavioral management, 136–137
behavioral therapy, medications compared to, 101–102
bipolar disorder, 42–43
birth
    ADHD in, 18
    premature, 20–21

brain
    ADHD and damage to, 13–14
    anatomy/function of, 8–10
    cognitive skills developed in, 19
    dopamine's function in, 64
    injuries to, 20
    neurotransmitters and, 10–12
    stimulants impacting, 52, 54–55, 64–65
    television impacting, 18

C

Catapres, 50, 63, 68
    pros/cons of, 98–99
caudate, 8–10, 13
celebrities, with ADHD, 14
Celexa, 95
cerebellum, 8–10, 13
children; *See also* adolescents
    with ADHD, 2
    ADHD outgrown by, 8
    disciplining, 135–136
    ear infections in, 21–22
    friendships and, 130–131
    iron-deficiency anemia in, 21
    parents discussing diagnosis with, 128–129
    stimulants refused by, 74–75
classroom adjustments, school
        accommodations and, 116–117
clinical trials, 97
clonidine (Catapres), 50, 68
    pros/cons of, 98–99
cocaine, 79
cognitive behavioral therapy, 132–133
cognitive skills, 19
college
    choosing, 124–125
    medications and, 83–85
    parents dealing with problems in,
        140–142
    preparing for, 123–125
    school accommodations in, 124
    stimulant abuse in, 92–94
    stimulants, adjustments for, 90–91
committee on special education (CSE), 117
communication
    problems with, 131
    school accommodations and, 117
    with teachers, 112
comorbidity, 37
    of conduct disorder with ADHD, 44
    learning disabilities and, 105
    of oppositional defiant disorder with
        ADHD, 44
    stimulant choices and, 94–95

compulsions, 41; *See also* obsessive-
        compulsive disorder
Concerta, 61, 62, 73
concussions, 20
conduct disorder, 37
    comorbid, 44
corpus callosum, 13
cross-over studies, 69–70
CSE. *See* committee on special education
culture, diagnosis and, 4–5
Cymbalta, 96–97

D

"DAMP," 105
DAT. *See* dopamine transporter
Daytrana patch, 61, 62
defiance, 44; *See also* oppositional defiant
        disorder
dependence, on stimulants, 78
depression, 25, 42, 68
Desipramine, 97
developmental language disorders, 21, 25
Dexedrine, 50, 54–55, 62–63
    methamphetamine compared to, 80
Dexedrine spantule, 62
Dextrostat, 62
diagnosis
    of ADHD, 3, 28–47
    age and, 4, 6, 8, 22, 36–37
    comorbidity and, 37
    culture and, 4–5
    history for, 28–29
    isolated behavior as, 23–24
    limited intellectual capabilities in,
        46–47
    medical tests and, 32–33
    in middle school, 36–37
    of mood disorders, 42–43
    of OCD with ADHD, 41–42
    over-, 35–36
    parents and children discussing,
        128–129
    parents notifying family and friends of,
        129–130
    personal agendas impacting, 3–4
    in preschool, 22
    quantitative questionnaires for, 4, 29
    quickness of, 31–32
    of tics, 39
    of Tourette's syndrome, 38–39
*Diagnostic and Statistical Manual of Mental
        Disorders*, Fourth Edition, Text
        Revision (DSM-IV-TR), 2, 40–41
    standards of, 3

dietary supplements, 102
disabled status, 120–121
disciplining, 135–136
disease, subclinical forms of, 37
disobedience, 27–28
disorganization problems, 107–108
doctors
    agendas of, 3–4
    choosing, 29–30
    personal visits to, 86–87
    types of, 30
dopamine
    addiction and, 79
    ADHD and transmission of, 11–12
    brain functions of, 64
    stimulants impacting, 54–55
dopamine transporter (DAT), 12–13
dosage, 57
double-blind studies, 69–70
driving
    self-control and, 138
    suggestions for, 139–140
"drug holidays," 89–90
drugs
    adolescents and, 137–138
    stimulants and, 85
DSM-IV-TR, 2
dyslexia, 21, 106–107
    definition of, 106

E

ear infections, 21–22
education; See also special education
    accommodations in, 114–117
    mainstream placement v. special
        placement, 111–112
    special benefits in, 35–36
EEG. See electroencephalogram
Effexor, 63, 96–97
electroencephalogram (EEG), 32
emotional functioning test, 34
environmental factors, 20
evaluations, 33–35
executive functioning abilities test, 34

F

family and friend notifications,
    129–130
family challenges, 133–134
family therapy, 134
Feingold diet, 102
fMRI. See functional magnetic resonance
    imaging
Focalin, 62

Focalin XR, 62
food intake, medication and, 73
friendships, 45
    children maintaining, 130–131
frontal lobes, 8–10
frontostriatal circuitry, 8
functional magnetic resonance imaging
        (fMRI), 32

G

gender, ADHD and, 26–27
gene pools, 5
gene therapy, 13
genes
    ADHD and, 12–13, 16–17
    discoveries with, 142
genetic proclivity, 16
growth, stimulants affecting, 69
guanfacine (Tenex), 50
    pros/cons of, 98–99

H

half-life, 98
head injuries, 20
heart, stimulants affecting, 65–66
heritability rate, 16–17
history (personal)
    confirming, 31
    for diagnosis, 28–29
homework problems, 109–110
hyperactivity–impulsivity, 5–6
    medication causing, 26
    symptoms of, 5–6
hyperkinetic disorder, 5; See also attention
        deficit hyperactivity disorder

I

IDEA. See Individuals with Disabilities
        Education Act
IEP. See individualized education program
impulsivity, 5–6
    symptoms of, 7
inattention, 5–6
    medication causing, 26
individualized education program (IEP), 117
    definition of, 118
    importance of, 118–119
    meetings of, 119–120
Individuals with Disabilities Education Act
        (IDEA), 35, 118
insecurity, 131
insomnia, stimulants and, 67–68
intellectual capabilities, limited, 46–47
intermediate-acting stimulants, 60

Intuniv, 50, 99
iron-deficiency anemia, 21
isolated behavior, diagnosis through,
    23–24

L

language disorders, developmental, 21, 25
Learning Centers, 124
learning disabilities
    comorbidity and, 105
    impact of, 104–105
    nonverbal, 105
legal counsel, special education and, 121
Lexapro, 95
limited intellectual capabilities, 46–47
long-acting stimulants, 60–61
Luvox, 95

M

magnetic resonance imaging (MRI), 32
mainstream education placement, special
    education v., 111–112
materials, school accommodations with,
    115–116
medical tests, diagnosis and, 32–33
medications; *See also* nonstimulants;
    stimulants
    behavioral therapy compared to,
        101–102
    college and, 83–85
    discontinuing, 84–85
    food intake and, 73
    holidays for, 87–90
    neurotransmitters, effects of, 63
    parents and decisions with, 75–81
    side effects of, 26
    timing beginning of, 59
    types of, 50
melatonin, 68
memorization problems, 106
metabolism, stimulants and, 57–58
Metadate OD, 62
methamphetamine, 80
Methylin, 62
Methylin ER, 62
methylphenidate, 50
middle school, diagnosis in, 36–37
mood disorders, 42–43
motivation problems, 137
motor problems, 38
MRI. *See* magnetic resonance imaging
MTA study, 51–52
Multimodal Treatment Study of Children
    with ADHD (MTA study), 51–52

N

neurological problems, 17
neurologists, 30
neurons, 10
neuropsychological assessment, 33–35
neurotransmitters
    brain and, 10–12
    definition of, 10
    nonstimulant medications effects on, 63
    stimulants effects on, 63–65
nighttime enuresis, 68
nonstimulants; *See also* selective serotonin
        reuptake inhibitors; serotonin
        norepinephrine reuptake inhibitors
    neurotransmitters, effects of, 63
    pros/cons of, 95–98
    types of, 95–102
nonverbal learning disabilities (NVLD), 105
norepinephrine, 55; *See also* serotonin
        norepinephrine reuptake inhibitors
    ADHD and transmission of, 11–12
note-taking accommodations, 115
NVLD. *See* nonverbal learning disabilities

O

obedience problems, 27–28
obsessions, 41
obsessive-compulsive disorder (OCD),
        26, 37
    ADHD diagnosis with, 41–42
occipital lobes, 9–10
OCD. *See* obsessive-compulsive disorder
Office of Disability Services, 124
oppositional defiant disorder, 28, 37
    comorbid, 44
organizational tutor, 110
overdiagnosis, 35–36

P

panic disorder, 40
parents
    agendas of, 3
    college problems and, 140–142
    diagnosis, family and friends notified by,
        129–130
    diagnosis of children discussed with,
        128–129
    disorganization problems and help from,
        107–108
    homework problems and, 109–110
    medication decisions of, 75–81
    support groups for, 134
    teachers informed by, 112–113

teachers selected by, 113
therapy guiding, 136
workspace efficiency and, 108
parietal lobes, 9–10
Parkinson's disease, 9
Paxil, 95–86
pediatricians, 30
personality changes, stimulants and,
66–67
personality disorders, 24
physicians. *See* doctors
placebo, 65
postsynaptic neurons, 11
premature births, 20–21
preschool
diagnosis in, 22
stimulants and, 71–72
presynaptic neurons, 11
private schools, special education and,
122–123
procrastination problems, 109–110
projective testing, 34
Prozac, 95
psychoeducational assessment, 33–35
psychologists, 30
assessments made by, 33–35
direct feedback from, 35
psychosocial problems, 17
psychotherapy, supportive, 132

Q

quantitative questionnaires, for
diagnosis, 4, 29
questionnaires, quantitative, 4, 29

R

reading disability, 106–107
rebound, 60
receptors, 11
Rehabilitation Act of 1973, Section 504,
120–121
restless leg syndrome, 68
risk factors, of ADHD, 16–22
Ritalin, 50, 62–63
Adderall compared to, 58
dosage of, 57
mathematics interest and, 54
overdose of, 74
overperscription/underperscription
of, 53–54
Ritalin LA, 61, 62
Ritalin SR, 62
rote information problems, 104, 106
rules, establishing, 135–136

S

safety, of stimulants, 50–53
SATs, 35–36
schedule, for stimulants, 87–90
school accommodations, 114–117
classroom adjustments and, 116–117
college and, 124
communication and, 117
materials and, 115–116
note-taking, 115
test-taking, 115
time and, 116
school notification, for stimulants, 83
Section 504 of Rehabilitation Act of 1973,
120–121
seizures, 25
selective serotonin reuptake inhibitors
(SSRIs), 63
side effects of, 96
types of, 95–96
self-control, driving and, 138
serotonin, 11, 55; *See also* selective serotonin
reuptake inhibitors
serotonin norepinephrine reuptake
inhibitors (SNRIs), 97–98
short-acting stimulants, 59–60
sibling challenges, 133–134
SNRIs. *See* serotonin norepinephrine
reuptake inhibitors
social impairment, 45
stimulants impacting, 72
special education
assessment for, 117
choosing, 113–114
committee on, 117
disabled status and, 120–121
legal counsel and, 121
mainstream education placement *v.*,
111–112
private schools and, 122–123
process of requesting, 117
"speed," 80
sports problems, 38
challenges with, 110–111
SSRIs. *See* selective serotonin reuptake
inhibitors
St. John's wort, 102
stimulants
abuse of, 78–79
addiction and, 75–81
advantages/disadvantages of, 56–63
alcohol/drugs and, 85
appetite suppression and, 66
brain and, 52, 54–55, 64–65

stimulants (*continued*)
    children refusing, 74–75
    cocaine compared to, 79
    college and abuse of, 92–94
    college and adjustments with, 90–91
    common, 62
    comorbidity and choosing, 94–95
    decision to take, 81–85
    dependence on, 78
    dopamine impacted by, 54–55
    duration of treatment with, 83–84
    effectiveness of, 55–56
    growth affected by, 69
    heart, effects of, 65–66
    insomnia and, 67–68
    intermediate-acting, 60
    long-acting, 60–61
    metabolism and, 57–58
    MTA study on, 51–52
    neurotransmitters, effects of, 63–65
    overdose of, 74
    overperscription/underperscription of,
        53–54
    personality changes and, 66–67
    positive response to, 55
    preschoolers and, 71–72
    rebound from, 60
    safety of, 50–53
    schedule for, 87–90
    school notifications for, 83
    serving, 72–74
    short-acting, 59–60
    side effects of, 65–69
    social impairment, effects of, 72
    tics/Tourette's syndrome and, 69–71
    time of year and, 59
    types of, 50
Strattera, 50, 63
    effectiveness of, 100
    side effects of, 101
striatum, 8–10
    anatomy of, 9
stubbornness, 44
study breaks, dealing with, 109
subclinical forms of disease, 37
substance abuse, 24–25
support groups, for parents, 134
supportive psychotherapy, 132
symptoms
    of ADHD, 7, 22–28
    age and change in, 22–23
    of hyperactivity–impulsivity, 5–6
    of impulsivity, 7
synapses, 10

T

teachers
    agendas of, 3
    communicating with, 112
    parents informing, 112–113
    parents selecting, 113
    style of, 106, 113
    warnings from, 81
team sports, 110–111
technological distractions, 108
teenagers. *See* adolescents
television
    ADHD and, 18–19
    brain and, 18
    cognitive skills impacted by, 19
temporal lobes, 9–10
Tenex, 50, 63
    pros/cons of, 98–99
test-taking accommodations, 115
therapy
    cognitive behavioral, 132–133
    family, 134
    parents receiving guidance through, 136
    reasons for, 131–132
    supportive psycho-, 132
thyroid problems, 25
tics, 30
    diagnosis of, 39
    stimulants and, 69–71
    vocal, 39
time, school accommodations and, 116
Tofranil, 97
Tourette's syndrome, 30, 37
    ADHD and, 38
    diagnosis of, 38–39
    stimulants and, 69–71
tricyclic antidepressants, 63
    advantages of, 97–98
tutor, organizational, 110

V

vitamin supplements, 102
vocabulary problems, 106
vocal tics, 39
Vyvanse, 61, 62

W

Wellbutrin, 63, 96–97
workspace efficiency, 108

Z

Zoloft, 95